Mind Over Platter ®

By Rosa Smith-Montanaro

"To be nobody but yourself in a world which is doing it's best night and day to make you everybody else means to fight the hardest battle which any human being can fight; never stop fighting."

e.e. cummings

This book is dedicated to my beautiful family Jerry, David, Rozetta and Regis. All of you have made it effortless to be myself, thank you. My prayer for you is that you too are free to be who God has created you to be.

Table of Contents:

The information in this book is not intended to replace the advice of your healthcare/medical professional and/or your nutritionist. We recommend that you consult with your doctor/health care professional prior to starting any weight management program.

The content of the material in this book is a result of The Mind/Body Institute, Mind Over Platter® and Rosa Smith-Montanaro, whose professional and personal experience as a hypnotist, NLP practitioner and weight loss coach has provided the inspiration for this publication.

It also represents years of research and study. Although the information in this book is based on a conglomeration of wisdom compiling books, tapes and educational seminars, the contents are the intellectual property of Rosa Smith-Montanaro, Mind Over Platter® and The Mind/Body Institute.

Although many the people mentioned in this book are real, their names have been changed. Some examples used are based on a "type" of person rather than an actual individual. Any resemblance is coincidental and not intended to reveal the identity of a factual person.

Acknowledgements

I, myself, usually skip this part of the book, but now realize that it takes a lot of people to complete a book. I would like to thank my wonderful community of choice.

Beginning with my husband "Jer", who has supported me while I have pursued my dream, and has loved me unconditionally since day one. I never have to be a "lone ranger" again. Thank you for taking such good care of me.

I could never have begun this without the ongoing support of my mentor "Clink", Clarence Thomson. Thank you for being my friend. I will forever be grateful to Rich Gardner for the first editing of my book, telling me my story had value.

I have been blessed with gentle spirited children who, for some reason, God has chosen me to guide in this world. I never imagined my reward would be so rich and fulfilling. You give me far more than I could ever give you.

Regis, you make me smile, your humor keeps me laughing. Your kindness melts my heart. Your loving presence brings peace to whatever you do. Your unconditional love has healed me in many ways.

Rozetta, who at only 17 years old, edited my entire book and has been my guardian angel. Thank you for telling me my story is AWESOME. You are a ray of light that fills the room with beauty and harmony. I am so proud of you. Your strength, wisdom and clarity are well beyond your years. I want to be like you when I grow up.

David, you have always been a calming force, so flexible, so accepting and so very playful. I appreciate how much you make us laugh and the joy you bring into our home. Simple experiences come alive when you are around. For this I am most grateful.

I have to thank my beautiful sisters: Nancy who's humor, talent and intelligence is a brilliant combination, and whose energy I marvel at. You are the most kind hearted person I know.

Anabel, who has embraced and supported me, I appreciate everything about you.

Jo-Jo who is not only my sister but one of my best friends, you are a blessing to me; your love has comforted me and reminded me that I am never alone. Just being with you makes me happy.

My sweet "baby" brother Dino who has always believed in me and affirmed my dream. I have such cherished memories our time together. My brother in-law(s): Pete, whose smile and positive attitude has always left me feeling energized and empowered. Billy for being so grounded, a voice of reason, and for bringing balance and humor to our crazy Italian family. Thank you for everything you have done.

My mother who is the reason for my deep faith in God, and who has taught me to have faith. My Uncle Joe and Aunt Anna for their unconditional love. And my father for telling me how much he loves me each time we speak.

I have to thank my friends: Terri Zbick, Joe Paglia, Bob Maynard, Jim Brault and Sue Wadja for their ongoing support and encouragement. My workout buddies: Lisa Wagner and Joanne Salva, the mornings are a blast! Wendy Brabon for helping me both personally and professionally. Ray Justice for coaching me through countless decisions. Also my many friends in the Greece community, especially from my Rotary club, Chamber of Commerce, BNI group and Greece Central School District.

I would also like to thank Angela and Helen from Angel Editing for their affirming feedback and excellent editing services. I have a special thank you for Rick McIntyre who is a great nutritionist and a wonderful teacher.

My dear friend from high school Jeannie Longchamps who first showed me what it feels like to be loved and valued with no strings attached. My very best friend Karen Magnuson who has been a blessing to me and has lovingly cheered me on. You are an inspiration to me. I really couldn't ask for better friends.

Most of all my beautiful clients and members of MindOverPlatter.com, it is you that motivates me most. I love you with my entire being. You have provided me with a purpose that humbles me. It is my honor to serve you, and I thank God for you each and everyday.

My Story: A Rose Blooms in the Desert.

"How I turned my biggest struggle into my biggest accomplishment."

Too often a new participant or client will look at me and say, "You don't know how I feel! You have no idea what I'm going through!" "This is hard for me" or "I will never be a size 4." They're referring to their weight, and the internal struggle and feelings of failure that go along with not being able to manage one's weight. These negative feelings affect our self-esteem and trickle into other parts of our life. We may feel unattractive and rejected by our spouse, when we may actually be pushing others away because we feel so badly about ourselves. When women at my seminars say to me, playfully, "I hate you, Rosa," everyone laughs and they look around and say, "Look at her; don't you just hate her?" They assume that because I look trim and petite that everything came easy for me. They are envious of what they see as my "perfect" life. They assume I had this handed to me, that I take it for granted. I have had this experience both personally and professionally.

I know what my clients are going through. As a matter of fact I know all too well what many women who feel inadequate are going through.

I work very hard now, and have since I was a young girl. I wasn't born into comfortable circumstances and I was barely accepted by the dysfunctional family I did have. We were very poor and I was raised on welfare and food stamps. There were times when the electricity was turned off and the phone disconnected. One time there was no food in the house and we ate whipped cream and bread sandwiches for dinner, since it was all we had. Santa didn't visit our home on Christmas except the year a stranger dropped off a box of food and gifts and said "Merry Christmas". It wasn't so bad being poor, but being treated like you are poor is humiliating. Most of my mother's family made insensitive comments within our hearing range. They would give us clothes for gifts because we needed them; I would watch my cousins get dolls and Barbies and pretend I wasn't disappointed.

I realized early on that if I wanted anything beyond food and shelter, I would have to go out and earn it. My father abandoned us when I was five years old.

My last childhood memory of him was him bringing me to school on my birthday, handing my teacher a cake and kissing me goodbye saying he will see me later. I didn't see him again until after my 21st birthday.

I had two little sisters, and my mother was pregnant with our brother. I adored my father and prayed every night that he would return. I wasn't sure why he left; all I knew was that I missed him so bad it hurt. I was sure he was unable to reach me. Growing up in the sixties and seventies, it was rare to have parents that were divorced. I was one of the only children in my class without a father.

My mother's brothers spent a lot of time in our lives. One of my uncles had an ongoing drug problem and would grow marijuana in our back yard and sell it out of our kitchen. I actually liked him and his friends when they were around. They were silly and playful. He wasn't much of a role model. Years later, when I became a teenager, he would smoke pot with me.

My favorite uncle has always been my Uncle Joe; he was compassionate and would help my mother in many ways. He would come to my open house and parent teacher conferences. I would pretend in my mind that he was my father. He was always sweet to me, my sisters, and brother. He would make Christmas special by spending time with us and bringing us a toy as a gift. I loved to brush my doll's hair, just like he brushed mine for me. I always felt loved by him.

In addition to my Uncle Joe, another person who just let me be a kid was my Aunt Santina. My Aunt Santina lived with us for awhile; she was my father's sister. I looked forward to being around her. She was very loving to us. She was very close to my mother. Even though my father left us, she would always remind me how much he loved me. Maybe because she loved me so much, I believed her. Aunt Santina was beautiful with her long dark hair and big brown eyes. She was half Italian and half African and had an exotic look. I remember her crying once because of a racial comment from one of my uncles; I climbed onto her lap and hugged her. I didn't know what the word meant but I knew it was hurtful.

My aunt moved away after a few years and we lost touch with her. Some of my favorite memories are with her.

My mother was raised by nuns in Italy and had low self-esteem. She herself had never felt loved and accepted and was emotionally unprepared to raise four small children on her own. She was often overwhelmed, depressed and angry about her situation. I always felt sorry for my mother, and tried to make her life easier by helping her take care of my siblings. On many occasions my mother would say "I can't buy enough for everyone (gifts, clothes, etc). The kids are little, so we have to take care of them, you understand." I would pretend it wasn't a big deal. I really loved my siblings and wanted them to have all of their needs met. Inside I felt sad and confused, "Why didn't she worry about me?" While on the outside I smiled and did what needed to be done. I was raised to be a caretaker and to worry about others more than myself.

Two things I recall Mom enjoying to do: reading a good book and cooking a big meal. She had a garden and with the little we had she would prepare some wonderful meals. When she had a few bucks we would take the bus to the public market and Mom would negotiate some good deals. She took pride in her cooking and it sure was a treat. I learned at an early age that food was love. Another reinforcement for this was on Sundays, a big day for the Italian culture. We would go down the street to my grandmother's house and she would make pasta and meatballs for us. It was the only time I could have soda pop, grandma would always have orange pop and sweets for us. I enjoyed the food and often ate far too much. This would become a life-long habit.

There are two things that you can count on in an Italian family: great food and a lot of drama. We had both.

When I was ten, my mother remarried an emotionally and physically abusive alcoholic who suffered from schizophrenia. I overheard his mother saying he was never the same since he returned from Vietnam. I can't imagine the demons he lived with; the rage and fury he expressed to our family has scarred us for life. I was at first excited to finally have a father, but was quickly disenchanted. On their wedding night he was so drunk he could barely walk.

He loaded all of us in his car and was going to drive us home. I was alarmed and frightened. Thank God his brother got in the car and insisted on driving. I would see him drunk, and unfortunately driving, on more times that I can count.

He was brutal to live with. He was verbally, physically, and emotionally abusive on a daily basis. He had a "clean your plate policy" that was never broken, forcing us to eat foods we didn't like. At the same time, if we upset him, which was easy to do being a kid, he would send us to bed without dinner. Sometimes my mother would later sneak food to us. He was a very unstable person in charge of the family and household.

He would hit us for inconsistent reasons. I would be washing the dishes debating with my sister and "pow", out of nowhere, my head was throbbing with pain and those black and white floor tiles would be racing toward my face. He didn't give warnings, just beatings. As the oldest child, I felt protective of my siblings and my mother. I would challenge my stepfather's judgment and his cruel behavior. It would result in him humiliating me either verbally by telling me how worthless I was, or with a spanking which would sometimes mean pulling down my pants and beating the daylights out of my bare bottom. He would say "If you would just shut your mouth; this wouldn't happen." But I couldn't shut my mouth, this wasn't fair and someone had to point it out. This has become my lot in life. For some reason I am the one who notices the emperor isn't wearing any clothes, and I need to tell everyone. They tell me to shut my big mouth and I can't. I wish I could, but for some reason it just fuels me further.

One time my siblings and I called the police because my stepfather was beating my mother. She was crying and pleading him to stop and he was yelling at her and hitting her in the face. I thought, "We have to save Mom." We ran down the street to our grandparents' home and called from there. After the police left, I was punished (sent to my room) and told by him, and my mother, to never do that again. My mother told me she deserved it, that she was wrong. I honestly didn't understand; a minute ago she was crying and now she loves him? I didn't get it. I thought something just isn't right here. Already, at this early age I was taught that my natural instincts were wrong. I was also learning that abuse is an acceptable way for a man to treat a woman.

As you can see, I was raised in a highly emotional household. My aunts, uncles, and grandparents would frequently argue. They would get into physical fights, throwing things and calling each other names and screaming hysterically. It was crazy to watch. My grandfather would throw the table upside down; my grandmother would be crying. A fight would break out between my uncles and my grandfather.

One of my uncles would hide us in a bedroom until it was all over. My grandfather was an alcoholic and had a violent temper. To this day my family still denies that he had a drinking problem.

Even though it would get crazy, I would often go to my grandmother's home to escape the madness of my own. When it was just her and my grandfather it was pretty calm. That was great until a family member who was visiting often asked me to go into the basement where he pulled down his pants (leaving his underwear on) and rubbed himself against me. He did this on a number of occasions. He would tell me this was our secret. I didn't understand what was happening but I felt dirty. I was never told this was inappropriate behavior but I avoided him based on my intuition.

My life was crazy. I grew up hearing my stepfather saying things like, "Rosa, you are so stupid; you will never amount to anything," or he would tell me how I wished I could be smart but never would be. One time my mother was hospitalized for her asthma and my stepfather told me "You are the reason your mother is sick again!" To his face I told him he was crazy and I couldn't make her sick, maybe it was his cat or dog? After all she is allergic to them. Boy did I get my butt kicked for being logical. But, inside I felt so guilty, "What if I am the cause? I do have a big mouth and I never know when to shut it. What if she dies because I have caused her so much stress?" That day when I spoke to my mother I told her I was sorry that she was sick and that I loved her. She told me she loved me too.

My mother was born and raised in Italy, and was a passive parent who wouldn't confront my stepfather. My stepfather had the freedom to hit me and send me to my room whenever he chose. I spent a lot of time in my room growing up.

When I became a teenager and began to look like a woman, he told me I was a tramp and couldn't be trusted with boys. He would accuse me of behaving like a whore. I would argue with him; then, for having such a "big mouth" he would hit me and send me to my room. None of what he said was true, but deep down inside I was afraid it might be. I would feel degraded from these encounters.

No matter how hard I tried to prove that I was a good girl, my efforts went unnoticed. I got As on my report card, and was elected Class President in eighth grade. I was always popular at school and well-liked by most people, but at home no one paid attention.

I made money babysitting at twelve years old and when I was fourteen, I had a paper route. I also worked part-time at the corner store. I was earning money to help out at home, and for some of the things I needed, but I still couldn't earn acceptance at home. My stepfather disliked me and was cruel to my siblings and to me until the day he finally left.

I found comfort in food. My mother grew many of her own vegetables and herbs, and was a great cook. Italian meals are generally festive times, and my mother would make them more special by preparing dishes that she knew were our favorites. My mother didn't say "I love you" much when I was growing up. Her way of expressing love was through food, and so she cooked for us.

During eight grade I was diagnosed with a severe case of scoliosis and required surgery. I would be in a body cast for the entire school year. This was traumatic for me but more so for my mother. Maybe due to the fact that all Italian mothers feel guilty for whatever happens to their children, she took excellent care of me. I required a great deal of assistance and she never complained. She went out of her way on a daily basis creating meals for me that she knew I would enjoy. It was then I realized that she really did love me and that maybe she loved me as much as my siblings.

My stepfather left when I was fifteen. He decided to pursue a career as an actor. He changed his name, packed his suitcases, took the family dog and was off to California.

He went promising to send for us once he was "discovered". During this time I was in a body cast recovering from my scoliosis operation and frankly I was glad to see him leave. He wasn't around that long, but he made an impact on our family that would last for years.

Shortly after he left, my body cast came off. I was enjoying simple pleasures like riding a bike, putting on my own shoes and taking showers. While I was loving life, Mom was missing her husband and she wanted to move to California to be with him. He told her I was too much to deal with and suggested I live elsewhere. By this time Uncle Joe and his wife, (Aunt Anna), lived in Arizona and she was seriously considering letting me live with them. I was devastated; I didn't want to move and cried for days. I was afraid I would never see my brother and sisters again. It was a very sad period of my life; I felt unloved and unwanted.

My mother came through for me, eventually divorcing him and we never heard from him again.

We had a neighbor who became very close to my mother during this time and encouraged her to turn to God and attend church. My mother has always read the Bible and had a strong faith in God, so it was natural for her to go in this direction. She quickly found a family at her new church and became "born again". It turned out to be a charismatic church that would stress the fire and brimstones of hell and the evils of this world. The pastor and his elders embraced my mother and we went to church three times each week. I was a teenager and behaving like one, talking back (big surprise), wanting to be with my friends and being boy crazy, which didn't go over well with the church.

My mother would turn to them for support and they told her that I was possessed by demons. Wasn't it obvious? I wore makeup, listened to rock music and had a boyfriend who was three years older than me. She allowed them to come to our home and destroy all of my records. When I arrived home from school I was furious and yelled at them. They then began praying and speaking in foreign tongues, attempting to exorcise the demons out of me. This scared the living daylights out of me. I was completely freaked out by the whole experience. I was petrified of demons as it was. I thought, "What if they really believed this? Could they hurt me to rid me of demons?"

I thought they were all unbalanced but I was powerless due to the fact that I was too young to legally leave home. This only confirmed that I couldn't trust my mother's judgment.

As a result of all of the criticism in my household I developed an attitude of "Well, if I am going to do the time, I may as well do the crime." I was no longer interested in being a good girl. I rebelled even more by running away from home a number of times. I would stay with anyone who would have me. I loved being away but worried about my siblings. I felt responsible to watch over them and protect them from the crazy life we were living. After a few rounds of this I eventually went home, allowed her and her friends to "save" me, was baptized (immersed) in water and even went to church camp. We celebrated this event by going out to dinner and having ice cream afterwards. This NEVER happened in my life before now. So food was my love and acceptance. It was my reward. I looked forward to my comforting, loving moments with food.

As a teenager I would often overeat until I felt stuffed and couldn't hold any more. Looking back on it, I can see how much sense it makes. I was starved for love and acceptance, and food filled the empty space inside me. As I became a young adult, I continued to find comfort in food, eating to get through the challenges and conflicts I faced. Then I discovered binging and purging, which meant I could eat whatever I wanted and purge it to feel better. This was a pattern that lasted for years. I was never obese, but I certainly did abuse food. It was my drug.

I had an unhealthy self-image and poor self-esteem. As a result, the attention that I received from my boyfriends was addicting to me. I once again tried very hard to gain the approval, this time from men. I made myself as attractive as I could, comparing myself to the women I saw in magazines and in the movies. In my mind I didn't measure up. It should be no surprise that I attracted men who would be emotionally and physically abusive. Because of my insecurity and my fear of abandonment I would cling to these relationships even though they were unhealthy and volatile. I recall my first boyfriend hitting me and as I was crying, he said "If only you would know when to shut your mouth, Rosa, I wouldn't get so mad.". I really believed it was my fault that I provoked men because of my personality.

I would question decisions that were made and the logic used. It ended up that most of my boyfriends cheated on me and what I was questioning them about was accurate. But deep down I feared that they were behaving this way because I was inadequate in some way. It just reinforced my belief that I was not good enough the way I was and I deserved what was happening to me.

Then I met Jeannie in high school. She was artistic, creative, smart and very witty. We couldn't be more different. She was French-Canadian, very proper and wholesome; I was Italian and flashy. We instantly became the best of friends; she was an angel for me. I never met anyone like Jeannie. She was normal; her family was warm and welcoming. Jeannie lived in the suburbs; I lived in the city. We did have one thing in common: our parents were divorced and our fathers couldn't stand us. We shared stories and related well to each other.

God brought her into my life to help me to grow. Jeannie was shocked at how my life was. She was the only person who ever told me I deserved to be treated with respect. She would complement me for being so responsible at home and for taking care of my siblings.

She would remind me that I was a teenager myself and should not be concerned with electric bills and school clothes for my siblings. Most of all Jeannie helped me to stand up for myself. If she saw a bruise on my arm, she would lecture me on how it was wrong to be hit. Jeannie opened my eyes. Even though it took me awhile to get it, her words rang in my head. I wanted to believe her and by listening to her, I was being reprogrammed in a positive way.

Her mother, Jacquie had the same impact on me. She loved me just as I was, with my makeup and eyeliner, tight clothes showing off my curvy body and sassy personality. She would affirm that I was special. Jacquie was an artist and dancer. She was very expressive and showed me an example of a mother who loved being a mother and expressed love and joy to her children. I thought Jeannie was the luckiest person in the world for having such a cool mom. I am fortunate for having such loving people in my life at a time when I needed someone to affirm that I was okay.

For affirmation, I would also turn to our neighbor Irene, a stay-at-home mom with three children. She too was very creative and a lot of fun. Irene liked to bake and many of my warmest memories are eating chocolate chip cookies at her house, especially on a snowy day. She believed children should be children and encouraged it. She had an open door policy and would welcome me and my siblings to come over whenever we'd like. Since I was older than her children, she would talk to me like I was an adult. She always praised my good grades, my accomplishments, and genuinely liked my company. I ran to her on many occasions to escape the madness. She never judged, just listened and praised me for being so mature and smart.

I couldn't wait to grow up and get on with my life. I knew I wasn't going through all of this for no reason. I didn't know what it was but I wanted to experience the world and find my place in it. I didn't know where I belonged, but I knew it wasn't where I was. When I finally had my chance and turned eighteen, I chickened out. My friends went to college; I went to work. Even though I knew I was intelligent and would thrive at a college, I couldn't do it. I didn't know who would help my mother and my siblings, so I chose working full-time, I often had more than one job.

As busy as I was, I was still in pain and trying to escape the terrible messages I had heard my whole life. I discovered drugs and partying.

After work I would go to parties until all hours; it was not a happy time in my life. I wasn't using good judgment and found myself in some pretty scary situations. The worst one being with a person who I agreed to go to a party with that turned into a nightmare. I ended up in a deserted wooded area with a very dangerous man who brutally raped me and threatened to kill me. This was the worst experience of my life. I was horrified and realized that if I didn't come home that night my mother might not report it for days. I thought, "I wasn't meant to die like this and end up as another tragic story in the newspaper." Even though I was not a religious person, I had faith that God had a purpose for me and that I would survive this ordeal. I believed the strength I had was divinely guided. Even though he repeatedly attacked me, I didn't panic, I was able to calmly convince him to let me go and I promised I wouldn't tell a soul. I never reported it; I told my sisters and a few of my closest friends. Years later he was convicted of rape and murder.

I wished I would have had the courage to have him arrested. I was so ashamed of my behavior and it reinforced my belief that I deserved what happened to me.

That event became a turning point for me. I decided my life would not be a waste and I would turn it around. I stopped partying and doing drugs. I decided it was time to change my ways.

At first, I attempted to escape my haunting memories by leaving my hometown. I ran away to Arizona to live with Uncle Joe and his wife. They never had children and encouraged me to come. They told me I always had a place to stay with them. I found comfort living with my aunt and uncle and felt safe. Since I was emotionally scarred and wasn't talking about it, I would stuff my emotions with food. I would binge and purge on a daily basis. I enjoyed cooking and since no one was home during the day, I would bake and prepare meals, all the while pigging out. I enjoyed finding a recipe and duplicating the results to serve my uncle and his wife. They liked my cooking and I enjoyed doing it, except I ended up gaining weight. I could barely fit in my clothes. I even had to cut the sides of my pants once. I suspect it was because I was feeling so out of control. I eventually got a grip on my eating and my weight returned to normal.

I realized that this wasn't solving my problems, so out of frustration I went to visit my best friend, Jeannie. She and her mother were staying with her aunt in San Francisco.

She invited me to spend the coldest summer of my life with them. My uncle and aunt were so disappointed that I didn't want to stay and make Arizona my new home. I spent a couple of months with Jeannie who had a job at a vegetarian restaurant and was able to get me hired there as well. It was a wonderful experience. She and I stayed up many nights talking and I confided in her about what happened to me that night. She told me that I didn't deserve to be treated that way and encouraged me to seek counseling.

Even though I loved being away and living in the West, I felt terribly guilty about leaving my siblings. I would call them to hear about how crazy it was at home and it just tore me up inside. I decided to return. I enrolled in school and I worked full-time.

I rekindled a relationship with the nicest man I had known in high school who I knew cared about me and would protect me. But I was in the relationship for all the wrong reasons so it didn't last. I feel badly for that kind man; he surely didn't deserve to be with someone as messed up as I was.

In January, on my twenty-first birthday I met a man and married him in December of that same year. I adored him, and he loved me. He was kind to me and very considerate. I was on my way; my dreams were all going to come true. The happy ending was finally mine! I was ready for this and optimistic. Unfortunately, I didn't realize that he, too, was an alcoholic, and we would experience some unpleasant confrontations that were, to me, painfully familiar. He had a violent temper and would blow up into a fit of rage with little warning. I became incredibly co-dependent in order to avoid his outbursts. I loved him very much and had a deep-seeded fear of abandonment. When we would argue, he would threaten to leave me. Many times he would disappear for hours or even days. I would be terrified, not knowing where he went and if he was okay. This was the most painful for me. The physical violence wasn't nearly as upsetting as being left; and I couldn't stand it. When he would return I would cry and promise to change. What a mess I was.

Because of his work we moved to California for two years and as much as I loved it, he hated it. Some of our worst "episodes" occurred there including him hallucinating and waking me up to tell me he discovered the anti-Christ. He was talking crazy and it scared me. I called a friend, thinking "What if he snaps?" My friend came over and prayed with me and as soon as we finished praying, my husband fell asleep.

We finally did move back home as a result of an argument where it ended with him packing his bags and going to the car telling me he was moving back East, with me or without me. I was pregnant with our daughter and couldn't bare the thought of my child growing up without a father. So I made the best of it by moving back home, 10 days after my daughter was born. I once again ate to cope with my life. I had gained nearly fifty pounds eating for two! This was a way to silence my unspoken fears. I knew my husband was a good man and that he meant well. I believed we could work through out problems if we tried hard enough.

So I went to counseling, group therapy, read self-help books, you name it, I tried it. He thought I was a control freak, and in retrospect I was. I wanted him to not kill himself. I wanted him to choose me over alcohol, and I wanted him to not lose his temper in the scary way he did.

I wanted to fix him and his drinking problem and absolutely believed I could help him. I also was convinced that if I could learn when to "shut my mouth" the violence would stop. But neither happened. I tried to be the "perfect" wife and mother and always felt as if whatever I did it was not good enough. I wanted the white picket fence. I wanted a husband, a home, a family, and eventually a career. I really thought it was possible, so I did everything within my power to "have it all". Boy was I exhausted.

This struggle continued for five years. Many times I thought we were on track with my husband abstaining from alcohol and long periods of time with no physical violence. Then when I least expected it I would discover an empty bottle hidden in the house or in the car. I would confront him and we would argue. I would stuff my emotions and fears with food. I even would binge and purge from time to time. I knew my life was out of control and there wasn't a thing I could do about it. I then had my second child, a beautiful baby boy! I had hoped my husband would want to discontinue his drinking since he had a son now. But his behavior only became more unpredictable. I admit I did put pressure on him to change and he didn't respond well to pressure. The violence returned and I was no longer able to avoid triggering his anger. It was at this time that I realized my life was never going to change.

I felt like I was on the verge of a nervous breakdown. I decided to attend a week-long seminar to escape my life and clear my head. During this time I grew very close to the other participants.

I shared my most intimate details including being raped. I experienced my biggest epiphany: I was good enough the way I was. I could cry if I felt sad and express my honest feelings and they still liked me. It never dawned on me that people would simply accept me just for being me. I also realized that I could not live the next seven years the way I just lived the last.

When I arrived home I told my husband that I didn't feel loved by him. That in order for me to please him I had to be quiet, tone my personality down and not be so enthusiastic. I told him that I liked me the way I was and that all I wanted was for him to quit drinking. He told me that I was right, he didn't love me and he wanted a divorce. Thirty days later he moved out.

This affirmed my hidden fear, that he could live with me or without me. I finally realized I needed to regain control of my life. I had two children and I was in the midst of a divorce. I was such an enabler that I consented to him filing for the divorce on the grounds of cruel and inhuman treatment in order to protect him. I was so worried about him getting through this that I never worried about myself. I just wanted to get on with my life. I thought: "Now, I get to live my life the way I want. I deserve to be happy." But, I realized I had some very negative programming to overcome. Since I didn't want to repeat the same mistakes and grow from my turbulent marriage, I decided to continue my work with counselors and therapists. I needed more help to overcome my painful memories and look at how they were contributing to the poor choices I was making.

Through my sessions with these professionals, I became aware of what happened to me as I was growing up. I was able to identify my feelings, and to see that they were valid. As a result, I learned to communicate how I was feeling in a healthy manner that honored myself and others.

I was encouraged to attend ALANON, because of my co-dependent personality and my past relationships with alcoholics. Through the twelve steps taught by ALANON, I embraced the concept of turning to a power greater than myself, God, a power to whom, if I entrusted myself, would strengthen me and my co-dependent nature. I had always believed in God but I had never surrendered myself to trust in God's will for me. I always thought all I needed was to take over and control the situation and it would be fine.

The problem is that we have little in life that we truly can control. Our ego drives the desire to control others and it usually leads to power struggles, not peace.

Armed with an awareness of my past and a new-found faith in my higher power, I was determined to move forward, to find true peace and happiness, and to replace the bad experiences I was now leaving behind me.

I longed to replace the painful memories and negative programming from my childhood with wisdom and insight. My quest continued in creating and manifesting a healthy and happy life. I still needed help.

I'd had an interest in the mind-body connection early on. All those times that, as a girl, I was sent to my room for punishment, I would read. I had started out reading romances, but soon found myself reading the likes of "The Power of Positive Thinking", "Sybil", and even "Psycho-Cybernetics". Maybe I thought that I was crazy, and I was looking for answers. Whatever my reason for reading those books, I discovered in them that the world I was living in wasn't the way it had to be. People in the real world could overcome things and they could lead productive and happy lives. So, as an adult, I again turned to self-help books and also sought out personal development seminars that would help me understand myself.

Tools that I found valuable in terms of building my self-esteem, my life as a whole, and changing my behavior, included Neuro Linguistic Programming, self-hypnosis, and Success Coaching.

Neuro Linguistic Programming, or NLP, taught me how language affects our minds and how empowering self-programming can lead to a positive attitude and resourceful solution-based thinking. It provided me with a process enabling me to make major shifts in my self-talk and self-image. I experienced transformations in my personal and professional life. As a metaphor, to signify my ability to overcome my past, I successfully attended a fire walk, walking barefoot over scorching hot coals without burning my feet. I knew my mind was powerful and this proved it to me. I acquired the ability to transform by neutralizing, even make positive, previously negative things. I remember one day, I decided to put my skills to work. While on the phone with one of my relatives, I was listening to her criticize me for not taking care of my mother.

I think she wanted me to provide my mother with a car or something of that nature. Previously my reaction would have been to feel defensive and angry then perhaps even resentful. I would think to myself: "Why couldn't she see that regardless of how much I do for my mother, no matter what I do, it isn't ever enough?" Then I would become depressed thinking "Most people my age have parents helping them; how will I ever make my way?" This used to infuriate me. But on this day I was, for the first time in my life, not concerned whether my relative understood me or even liked me. By applying an NLP technique, while on the phone, our whole conversation instantly shifted.

This time I actually felt love for her. I understood she'd had a hard life, having been born in a foreign country (Italy), and had suffered some significant cultural limitations. I was able to thank her for calling me, tell her I loved her, and hang up. I realized I didn't feel any negative feelings about what just happened. I felt a sense of peace! I recall doing the victory dance in my kitchen, celebrating my new-found freedom.

Self-hypnosis gave me the ability to reprogram my subconscious mind. Once I understood that all habits and beliefs are unconscious, I learned how to change negative beliefs about myself into positive, empowering beliefs. I was able to heal so much of my pain from my childhood using self-hypnosis. I did it using visualization techniques, which have helped me transform my life. It is my belief that the subconscious mind is divinely attuned. It can easily access all of the resources we need to accomplish our goals. The only thing holding me back was that my conscious mind was too busy; it wasn't listening to the wisdom of the higher consciousness. God easily communicates with the subconscious mind through our intuition. Self-hypnosis quieted my mind, gave me a positive focus, and literally redirected my brain, guiding it toward the goal that I desired. I am living proof that this is true.

Success Coaching taught me a new way of living. It introduced me to the concept of aligning my life with my values and living a life that has purpose. With a coach I was able to discover my truth, my inner wisdom. From this awareness I created an action plan that honored me.

This model is pro-active, as well as co-active. For myself, I liked working with a coach who asked powerful questions and elicited what was in my heart. We focused on what I wanted to manifest and was in my best interest.

Together we created an action plan and my coach held me accountable to follow through. I have written this book from a coach's perspective; using the same approach has helped me and I have used it with my personal clients.

I also began studying nutrition and herbal supplementation. I have a deep respect for the old Eastern ways of looking at things, and I've been influenced by watching my mother grow herbs and vegetables, and experiment with natural remedies.

Since weight management is multifaceted, the mind is a big component to success, but the body must be in balance as well. Insulin must be managed. In my family, most of my relatives are overweight, have diabetes, high blood pressure and heart disease. I knew I needed to start early if I wanted to prevent these medical problems. So I studied how to prevent, even reverse these problems with a proper nutrition and a healthy lifestyle. By living this way, the side benefit is weight loss!

Through the power of self-hypnosis, NLP, and the basic principles of Success Coaching, I was able to make major changes in the way I perceived my life and my experiences. I felt more optimistic, empowered to create a whole and balanced life. As I grew closer to God, I came to understand with total and complete certainty that God is connected to all of us. God loves and accepts each of us. We have a potential that we can reach. God gave us brilliant minds; through Him we are able to heal ourselves emotionally, and reach that potential, just by using our minds properly. My relationship with God has given me peace, hope, and courage. I am truly blessed in every way. Not only have I maintained my ideal weight for over eight years but more importantly, I am happy.

I enjoy loving and authentic relationships with my family and friends. I have amazing children; I am thankful to God for allowing me the privilege of being their mom. I have remarried and have a sweet husband who not only loves me, but is in love with me. He is loyal and committed to our marriage. He supports me and finds my "big mouth" and expressive personality delightful and even amusing at times.

I am proud of my first husband, he has not had a drink many years, and we have successfully co-parented our children. My mother and I are very close. I love her so much and we say "I love you" every time we speak. She is a blessing to me and my children. I now have a relationship with my father; I know he loves and cares deeply about me. He is a loving grandfather. I am surrounded by nurturing and loving people.

I am now living a life that is based on my values and my life's purpose.

I had asked myself many times over the years, "If I could do something for the rest of my life, what would it be?" Now, the answer was suddenly clear. I would take what I learned from this turbulent, yet wonderful experience and help others.

I had achieved such a sense of freedom and joy from letting go of all of my early baggage and replacing it with empowering beliefs that I wanted to tell the world, to help others achieve what I did. I decided to focus on weight, since I used food to deal with my emotions and life's struggles. I could strongly relate to how it felt to not manage one's weight. I wanted to combine the techniques that had helped me: NLP, hypnosis, and Success Coaching, to help others find peace and happiness and even become "naturally" thin.

Just how would I take what had once been my biggest struggle and make it my calling, to help others?

In one of the trainings I had taken, I was given the assignment of writing an extensive paper. I chose to outline a process I would use to help people lose weight. My program had twelve sessions and incorporated what I learned in NLP, Success Coaching, and self-hypnosis. I now call it Mind Over Platter®. I based it on what I learned about the mind/body connection, that how the mind thinks and believes has an impact on our lives. We choose to take action as a response to our thoughts and beliefs and are unconsciously literally co-creating our reality. This experience then reinforces our beliefs which then influence our thoughts, thus creating a self-fulfilling prophecy.

If this was true, then all I needed to do was study a naturally thin person (one who would gain weight if they overate, but successfully maintained an ideal weight). Discover what they think and believe is true about food and their bodies. Observe their habits and behavior. Then compare this to how a chronic dieter (one who struggles and is overweight), thinks, believes and behaves.

Once I made these distinctions, I could actually duplicate the naturally thin person's mindset and teach it to a chronic dieter, pointing out the habits and beliefs that they needed to change. I found this to be easier than I had imagined as naturally thin people have similar habits. Being a chronic dieter, I tested my theory on myself and it worked! Just by following these principles I lost 30 pounds.

My teacher was so impressed with my program that she began referring clients to me. Satisfied clients began referring others. When I started seeing the power of the shift in my clients' thinking and actions, I developed and trademarked Mind Over Platter® into an actual seminar, and started teaching it at various businesses and at local schools. My clients insisted I record self-hypnosis sessions and my seminars on CD to support them. Many of my clients would listen to the CD when they were out of town and shared them with their friends. Numerous people have credited listening to the self-hypnosis CDs for helping them to lose up to 50 pounds.

To help more people and to reach people who couldn't attend my seminars, I created a virtual weight loss coaching program, www.MindOverPlatter.com.

This program had everything I used to help my clients and students to lose weight, all available 24 hours a day, 7 days per week on the Internet. I added self-hypnosis sessions on the website, an outline of my coaching process and many tools including an automated food journal for members to track what they ate. This program has proven to be successful and even earned me the award of e-Business Executive for 2004.

I am not a doctor, nutritionist, or psychologist. I am a woman who has traveled a journey through adversity and some painful memories. When people say "Do you have a Master's degree?" I say, "My life is my Master's degree!" I was able to take bad programming and transform my life. I went from believing that I had no value and would never amount to anything to having a pretty great life. All areas of my life have improved; my body, my self-image, self-esteem, relationships, even my business has grown in wonderful ways.

If I can do it, you can do it. I want you to think of me as your personal weight loss coach. I have a wealth of knowledge and experience to share with you. Are you willing to take it and apply it to your life? One small change can make a remarkable difference in your life. I didn't change overnight; it took years. Growth, whether it is emotional, spiritual, or personal is a process that feels like a spiral. You feel like you are going round and round with little progress, but when you look back the spiral is actually going up, having advanced you further than you realized.

The problems you once used as an excuse to hold you back are surfacing less and less. The more you apply what I am teaching in this book, the smoother the journey will be. I understand this process; there is no shortcut, my friend. The only way through it is through it, but you are not alone. I am here beside you, guiding you every step of the way. I want what is best for you, for your highest good. I thank God for bringing us together; it is my honor to serve you.

Good luck and God bless you, my dear friend.

Your faithful weight loss coach,

Rosa

How to Use this Book

I am a natural student; I thrive on learning. When I hear an interesting new concept, my reaction is always, "How does it relate to my life?" If I can integrate it into my life, starting today, great! If I can't, then it may only make for an interesting discussion.

I am also a natural teacher; I enjoy sharing. To be able to share with you what I've learned makes the experience twice as valuable. I have written this book with you in mind as my coaching client. It contains practical concepts that can be integrated into your life, starting today. You'll want to practice them, not merely discuss them.

When I decided to remarry, I picked up a wedding planner from the magazine rack at the supermarket. You know the kind; they cover every detail in the planning of a perfect wedding. I found it very useful and referred to it often. Because I spent time planning my wedding, it actually did go perfectly. At the time I was just starting my coaching business. I asked myself, "What if I could map out a plan and system like this for my business?" Up to this point I had been flying blind in terms of reaching larger numbers of clients and growing the business. So I created a series of strategies, action items, milestones, and checklists. It was extremely helpful; my business did a one-eighty. My clients thrived and my practice grew, in the quality way I wanted it to. With that plan, I became successful.

When I wanted to help my clients lose weight, I did the same thing. I created a plan, a series of action items and checklists. Besides the plan, I included two very important tools, the same ones I had used throughout my life, especially when I felt my life was out of control. Those tools were journals, one for recording the food I ate each day, the other for writing down my thoughts and feelings.

Thoughts would surface, such as one day realizing that my mother had always used food to say, "I love you" to me. Even after I was married and she came to visit, she would bring huge pans of traditional Italian dishes – cooked with pasta, sauces and meats. I couldn't eat everything, but I couldn't throw them out either because my mother made them for my family and me. So I would let them sit in the refrigerator until they spoiled and it finally made sense to throw them away.

I continued to allow my mother to do this for some time, and let them go to waste. Finally I spoke to her about it, saying "Mom, please don't bring so much food, we won't eat all of it." This was a very big deal for me, for us. We both grew from this, communication. I learned from realizing that I accept her cooking in place of her saying she loves me, and she in having to show me she loves me without food. Insights like these I call epiphanies. They are the realizations, the light switch turning on in your mind. As a result of this epiphany my mother and I have a loving relationship and now say "I love you" to each other every time we say goodbye.

My clients found by journaling both what they feel as well as recording their food intake to be insightful. They began to have their own epiphanies. To begin your own personal journal, just use any composition book. As far as a food journal goes, you can write down what you eat in a book or use an automated journal online. Both are available on MindOverPlatter.com.

This book is more than a weight loss program. It is your planner. It will provide you with numerous opportunities to journal, contemplate, and recode your epiphanies. Please use it as your coaching journal. As you will see, I will ask you to take action at the end of many of the chapters in the form of a thought-provoking assignment.

Although the sequence of each chapter is intentionally arranged in an order to most benefit you, each chapter is independent within itself. I have written it so that you can later refer to the areas that most fit your needs. You will intuitively know which chapters you need. I suggest reading the entire book, then going back to the chapters as you need them.

I have chosen to divide the book into two parts: Mind and Body. The first half is for your mind, the second for your body (beginning with "Your Diet Personality"). I did not discuss the actual food plan until later because I would like for you to have your head in the right place. I believe when your thinking is clear anything will work, when it is confused, nothing will work. I also know that when you want to lose weight, you want to get started while you are motivated to begin. You can immediately begin applying the suggestions for how to change the way you eat, **while** you read about how to change the way you think.

This is why I would like for you to form a Mind Over Platter Weight Loss Support Team. This will empower you to lose weight while you reprogram your mind.

The food plan works; you will lose weight, but if you want to keep it off then please follow through on the rest of the program. This will *train your brain to think like a naturally thin person.*

I encourage you to make a commitment to yourself that you will read this book and use the tools that I am sharing with you, this can be a life changing experience. I will also periodically highlight a "Thinking Thin Thought". This is like an affirmation; repeat it to yourself daily until it starts to integrate into your life. If it resonates with you then it means that you will benefit from bringing the new belief into your awareness.

When forming a Weight Loss Support Team, I strongly suggest you find friends who want to make their health a priority. Make a commitment to support each other. Meet weekly and complete the assignments. Discuss the "Thinking Thin Thought" statements. I would also recommend you share your food journal with each other. Being accountable and having support will dramatically increase your success. People who join our program with a friend lose almost twice as much weight as people who go it alone.

I wish you well. My prayer for you will be, like it has been for thousands of clients, that you nourish your mind, body, and spirit. That you experience enlightenment, and you integrate your epiphanies into your being, allowing you to manifest who you know in your heart you were meant to be. You are a divinely guided, wonderful person. You deserve to feel loved, you deserve a healthy body, and you deserve to be happy.

Look at this journey as a process, like planting a garden. Your garden is your mind. You plant seeds (suggestions), pull the weeds (negative beliefs), provide fresh water (empowering beliefs), and expose it all to sunlight (positive, supportive people). It takes time, patience, and persistence, and in time, your garden will flourish.

Your Assignment:

- Start a Food Journal
- Start a Feelings Journal
- Form a support team (4-8 people)
- Commit to meet weekly.

When you meet with your team:

- Weigh in privately.
- Record your weight privately.
- Discuss the assignment or chapter you are reading.
- Share your food journal with someone.
- Discuss how you felt saying the "Thinking Thin Thought" statement.
- Listen to a visualization CD (Imagine Yourself Thin).
- Offer suggestions and encouragement.
- Discuss what you will commit to over the upcoming week.
- Celebrate your success!

I have provided forms on www.MindOverPlatter.com under the "Weight Loss Programs" link. Entitled: "Start your own Weight Loss Support Team"

Weight Management is a Lifestyle Not an Event

You are not alone in your weight loss journey. I invite you to consider me as your personal weight loss coach. I am your partner in success. *"Weight management is a lifestyle not an event."* My intention is to be your coach every step of the way.

I am committed to teaching you about the art and science of weight management. This is an integrated approach to weight management; by that I mean mind, body, and spirit.

- Mind: change the way you think.

- Body: diet, change the way you eat.

- Spirit: healing is a spiritual process.

To enjoy a healthy lifestyle you must first create a healthy mind as well as body. When you accomplish this you will find a path of inner peace and desire to connect to others in a meaningful way, thus honoring your spirit. I believe God wants all of us to live in harmony with each other and to do so in healthy bodies. There is a lot that we can accomplish in our lives and we need strong healthy bodies and minds to accomplish it.

I am equally committed to inspiring and empowering you to take back control over food by enlightening you about the profound impact of your thoughts on your body. By reading this book and applying these principles, you will have a clear understanding of how powerful your mind is and how you can use this insight and power to achieve anything in life you desire, including a naturally thin lifestyle.

I want to congratulate you for taking the first step to changing your life. You are reading this book and that is a HUGE step. You will be planting some powerful seeds in your mind. I hope you will take action on the suggestions. As I stated earlier, you must change the way you think; create a naturally thin mindset.

What do I mean by mindset? Whatever you believe is true for you, is true for you. It is all a matter of perception. People who do not struggle with their weight, whether they are overweight or underweight, subconsciously have a belief system that supports the body they live in.

After you've changed your mindset, you can change your behavior by creating some empowering habits. Additionally, you will need to change your lifestyle by creating a healthy and fit body. And you will be grateful for the wonderful lessons you have learned, and taught yourself, along the way.

I want to begin by reminding you that you are a special and incredible person. You have a body but you are not only your body. You are far, far more than your body. It is my belief that you are already whole and amazing exactly as you are at this very moment. Nothing can change that. I challenge you to accept it as the truth and watch how your life changes.

When you are not happy with your body, it is easy to lose sight of how delightful and truly magnificent you are. It becomes even more difficult to realize your highest potential when your body lacks the energy necessary to carry out your life the way that you want to.

Many people say things like, "I will like myself when I lose weight," or "I wear a size 6." Then they may go on a drastic diet telling themselves that once they reach their goal things will change.

Thinking like that can be a waste of our precious time. Why? Because of our egos. The ego is self-centered and is never happy. The moment that we accomplish a goal, like losing weight, our ego will convince us that what we have still isn't good enough. We raise the bar. We decide to change our mind once again, and shoot for more. We are all guilty of this.

If you are truly going to savor the moment and enjoy reaching your goals, you have to first learn how to change the way you think. Otherwise, you will never be happy, with your weight or your body. I will show you how to change the way you think.

Start liking yourself today. When I first set out to lose weight and take back control over my life, I began each day by saying, "I love and accept myself as I am right now." I would say it every single day, over and over again.

Did I believe it? No.

Did it help me? Yes. I stopped focusing on the bad things that I perceived about myself. You may or may not see a difference right away, but the positive self talk will bubble up in other parts of your life.

Why wait until tomorrow? Start today. Make a conscious decision to like yourself right now, or at least be willing to try. Trust me, it is a far more peaceful journey and sweeter victory when you love yourself without conditions.

My dream for you is that you will come to a place of self-appreciation and a deep sense of love for who you are on the inside. You are divinely created. You deserve to claim that truth and honor it. Once you do this, then the outside will follow. It always does.

How do I know? Because I have been there. For years I had gained and lost weight. I came to a point where I hated my body. It was affecting my attitude and my life. Back in 1996, when I was preparing to attend an extensive training seminar in St. Louis, I had reached a major turning point in my life. As I sat in my hotel room and looked at myself in the mirror I was disgusted with my body. I felt fat and unhealthy. I only packed bulky sweaters and oversized shirts to wear. To make matters worse it was a hot June and I was so uncomfortable. I actually heard my self saying, "Look at you, Rosa. You are gross!" I began to realize that all of the negative messages that I was sending myself couldn't be good for my body.

I was 30 pounds heavier than my current weight and I felt desperate. I began to see how hurtful my thoughts were. It was at this moment that I decided to stop tormenting myself and to do something. I made a decision to learn to like myself as I was, and to practice gratitude in my life. I thanked God for what I did have, a healthy body, free of illness. I realized I could be stuck with my body for the rest of my life, so I decided to make the best of it and make peace with it. I thought, "Rosa, the worst thing that can happen is you spend the rest of your life at this weight. Relax. If the worst thing to happen to you in life is to remain at this weight, you are pretty lucky."

Here is the interesting part. Once I made this decision, God put people in my path to help me manifest self-love and acceptance. It was at this seminar in St. Louis that I would meet my mentor, "Clink", who is an expert in the Enneagram. He agreed to teach me about the Enneagram and we still communicate on a regular basis.

Clink, being a former Catholic priest, has a loving presence. He has shown me what it feels like to be loved and accepted for doing nothing. Not a single thing. Do you know how foreign that was to me, to not earn love and acceptance? It was radical, but he reinforced it time and time again with his kind words of wisdom. He would remind me "God loves you, Rosa" and "I for one love you just the way you are." With his example and my new outlook I began to see myself differently.

Then something happened! I started to be nicer to myself, sending myself positive messages instead of negative ones, such as "God loves me as I am…so should I!" I began to feel happier, more peaceful. I even began to lose weight! I lost 30 pounds, achieving my ideal weight, and have kept it off.

In my practice as a Weight Loss Coach, I shared these insights with my clients and it began to have an impact on them as well. They saw that by learning to love themselves just as they were, the very least that would happen was that they would find peace with themselves. They didn't feel that sense of urgency that comes when we place the completion of weight loss, success, or any other conditions on our self-love.

Then, they also began to experience change. They began to glow because they were honoring their true selves, just as they were. They ate healthier foods and exercised more. Little by little, the weight came off for them as well.

I was seeing first-hand that my experiences and beliefs were correct. What had worked for me was working for my clients. There are few moments in your life when you make a decision that can change your destiny. I believe that this is one of those moments. Don't put it off another day. Today is the day to take back control over your life, and over food.

The Mind:

Self-Love and Acceptance

Imagine not being preoccupied with your weight. Imagine having the patience and confidence to diligently and consistently advance in the direction of your healthy body. Imagine being free from stress and doubt. Let yourself wonder what it would be like to lose weight without deprivation, no self-punishing diets, no self-defeating thoughts.

The foundation of empowerment, the path to creating true life-long change, is in this kind of self-love and acceptance. However, it may not be the change that you expected. Achieving self-love in itself may not make you thin, but it will give you something more precious. Self-love will change the reason why you do what you do. When you love yourself, you are grounded in a position of power. No matter what occurs in your life, you will be certain of your value and worth as a person. You will be filled with a sense of peace, knowing that you are a unique, special, divine being.

Once you are able to truly love yourself, you will be happy with your body regardless of whether you lose weight or not. Either way, you win! Some people fear that they will not be motivated to lose weight after applying this mindset.

My experience and that of many of my clients is in fact the opposite. Pure motivation and optimal results come from a sincere desire to take your life to a higher level, not from a sense of self-hatred. Sure, you can be driven from anger and fear, but you won't have peace. Think about the person who uses anger and fear to motivate themselves, radically starving themselves in a self-punishing way. They are uneasy and have high levels of stress, which isn't healthy for their body. Then think of the person who is beginning to appreciate and love themselves with a much more reasonable approach. It may include a walking schedule, nurturing, not starving their body, and accepting that a change in attitude and achieving results will take time.

When you accept yourself with love, you will free yourself from what the world wants from you. Instead you will discover who you are, and what you want for yourself. It's like taking yourself by the hand and lovingly leading yourself to a healthier body instead of dragging yourself, heels dug into the ground, up a hill.

To start this process, repeat this affirmation daily: "I love and accept myself exactly as I am." The harder this is to say, the more you need to say it!

Affirming self-love alone can completely change your life. As you repeat this affirmation, take a moment to envision yourself in a healthy, fit, attractive body. Allow your mind to settle on this image, and believe in your heart that this is really you. Take a moment to be with this wonderful, delightful, happy person – yourself.

What does it feel like to say these words and see this image? Is it difficult to envision? That's okay, just keep saying it every single day until you automatically start thinking, "Yes, I do love myself, I am great!"

Martha's Struggle:

When I first met Martha she wanted to lose 100 pounds. She was beautiful, her skin was smooth and youthful, and she had a bright smile that would light up the room. She had a great sense of humor and could make people laugh with almost no effort. I thought she was great. When I asked her to begin to say, "I love and accept myself exactly as I am," she couldn't do it. She would begin to cry. I assured her that she needed to be willing to say these words that I have seen change people's lives, including my own. I asked her to agree to do it daily, for a week, until our next appointment. When she came back into my office, I already saw a brighter, more peaceful Martha. She hadn't lost much weight but she was feeling so much happier that she actually looked thinner, less overwhelmed by her physical body.

Martha had always been told, as many women growing up, "You would be so pretty if you just lost weight." And she believed this. In fact, for years she had "filtered" for that statement. By "filtered," I mean she was unconsciously seeking out people who would say that as an affirmation that it was true. As a result, she was postponing feeling pretty until she lost weight. I not only encouraged Martha to say, "I love and accept myself exactly as I am," I also asked her to add, "I am an attractive woman."

While Martha was coming to see me, she was also dating. Several weeks into our working relationship – she had lost twenty pounds.

Martha and her boyfriend were talking casually when he made the comment "You're pretty when you lose weight." She had an epiphany; she was already pretty and made a decision in that moment. She was too pretty for him and decided to break up with him and never look back. She realized he had just told her the exact same thing that she had been telling herself, and believing, for years! But now she could rewrite that belief, she was already an attractive woman with or without the weight.

Martha was happy and felt successful. I saw a difference in her from Day Two. She was feeling happier and enjoying her new experience before the first five pounds were shed. That is the true success, when you feel comfortable in your own skin. She did end up reaching her goal, but the real victory came when she decided she was worthy of love and acceptance.

You have a choice: You can lose weight the old-fashioned way, forcing yourself to follow a diet and telling yourself you are fat each time you look in the mirror. Or you can say, "Hey, I am pretty special and I deserve to be healthy." I've done it both ways. The first path hurts; the second is joyful. The path of choice is self-love and acceptance.

I understand how difficult it is to overcome challenges, especially when you may have had a lifetime of negative programming. When you begin this journey old, unpleasant, negative beliefs may pop up. Don't be discouraged.

I have had to overcome so much to find inner peace and a strong sense of self. This was not an easy process for me either, but it is worth it. I already mentioned in the introduction that my father walked out on us when I was five, and things went downhill from there, at least for the duration of my growing-up years. I heard some pretty negative messages about my worth from the adults around me. I can't remember how many times my stepfather told me how stupid I was and what a loser I was.

It isn't surprising, then, that I found the affirmation, "I love myself," most challenging at first. I kept hearing the self-talk in my mind with another message, "Yeah – right – who are you kidding Rosa?" My challenge came from a deep fear that I was not worthy or deserving of love and appreciation. As I explored where this was coming from, I had to face the painful question, "How can I be lovable when my father left me?" "How can I be loveable when my stepfather said all of those terrible things to me and my mother didn't say anything to disagree?"

I unconsciously believed the messages I was hearing from my past, even though I knew consciously that they were not true. I knew that my mother was afraid of my stepfather and didn't agree with his actions. But unconsciously I feared that she did.

You can change negative programming. I did it and I know you can as well. In this book you will learn multiple ways to change the way you think. To start with, when you hear negative self-talk, stop and tell yourself, "Snap out of it!" and immediately think a positive, empowering, loving thought instead.

Look for examples/signs of being loved:

> ➢ *"My children love me."*
> ➢ *"I have friends who love me."*
> ➢ *"There are a lot of people who do care about me."*
> ➢ *"These people see good qualities in me."*

We should not have to look to external reinforcement for self-affirmation; right now we are at a crucial point, the beginning of your involvement in this program. You likely have a belief system that needs to be changed. You need to build positive references to replace old ones that you now realize are negative and haven't worked for you. You need these new references right now to affirm that you are, indeed, lovable. In other words, you need to filter in the proper external messages, until you can establish your own new internal references.

My own "unlovable" issues centered around being abandoned by my father, then being mistreated by my stepfather. So when, for example, I thought about my biological father not loving me, I replaced it with, "My heavenly Father adores me. I have a Father who loves me more than I could ever imagine. There is nothing that I can possibly do to change that; I am totally loved by my real Father, who will never leave." Because I believe this, God sends me constant reminders of wonderful people who love me just the way I am, such as my mentor, my editor, my children, my best friend, and my husband.

Your Assignment:

As you follow this program daily, give yourself the gift of spending just a few moments each day envisioning yourself in this incredibly healthy body, and repeating your self-love affirmation. Do this every morning as you wake up and every evening before you go to sleep.

Thinking Thin Thought:

Repeat this affirmation until it becomes a belief for you:

"I love and accept myself exactly as I am. I am worthy and deserving of love."

Attitude of Gratitude

Self-love and acceptance occurs naturally when you experience life from an attitude of gratitude. This is an important concept that cannot be reinforced enough. Gratitude, say it out loud, "gratitude." How do you feel? What other words come to mind? You might be thinking of words like thankfulness, appreciation, and grateful.

Thinking of these words leads to feelings of love, self-acceptance and inner peace. You might be seeing a trend here with how I approach weight loss. It always comes back to changing your perception, which will change the way you feel, which changes the way you think; resulting in changing your behavior.

What do you have to be grateful for? A lot! I had a client who was in the last stage of her weight loss program; she had twenty pounds to go before her goal. She just couldn't seem to do it. She felt overweight, her clothes were still too tight, and it was affecting other areas of her life. One day, I had just returned home from a funeral. My teenage daughter's friend's mother had died. My client called, saying the twenty extra pounds were ruining her life. Now, I had just returned home from seeing two teenage boys bury their mother. My perspective was how those boys wished they had a mother who was carrying an extra 20 pounds. I told my client that as long as she was alive and healthy, she had something to be grateful for. She needed to start appreciating her own life, by finding reasons to be happy. I told her, to begin her day expressing gratitude. It can be as simple as applying lotion to your skin in the morning and thanking that part of your body for being healthy.

Gratitude is how I transitioned from frustration to appreciation of my body. You can transform your life by living with an attitude of gratitude. Think about how much your perspective can change just by the way you look at a given situation.

I used to think to myself, "Life isn't fair; I gain weight so easily!" Then I felt angry. I actually felt betrayed by my body. If I ate French fries, I gained weight. It wasn't a gluttonous act. Other people ate them and it didn't bother them, yet for me, I gained a couple of pounds and had to work it off. "It isn't fair!" I would say. Then I would feel deprived and I would focus on the food I couldn't have. This led to envy, even resentment of people who could eat fries and not gain weight.

This pattern of thinking didn't work in helping me regain control over food. It gave power to the food. It kept me stuck in a place that I didn't want to be. That can be a dangerous place if you stay there too long.

When you feel frustrated or angry and don't address it, then resentment is sure to follow. This is really important to notice in your life – how do you feel when you have unresolved anger and resentment? Depression, is also known as anger turned inward. I see women and men in my office who are overweight and depressed. Untreated depression can bring you down a slippery slope very quickly. It is normal to feel sad, and discouraged for a few hours which is different than long periods of sadness, despair or feeling hopeless which is a sign of depression. It will immobilize you and rob you of the joy in your life.

Don't let something as manageable as weight and food intake be the source of depression. You can lose weight and you can take back control over food. People become depressed because they gain weight and then they eat to help them cope with the depression, only to cause them to feel more resentment fueling their depression. Then they eat to cope with the depression, they then gain weight. It is an endless cycle and can be successfully avoided.

I speak from experience. I have worked with thousands of people. I have seen the pitfalls. They think the weight's the problem, the source of their depression. That may or may not be true. My experience tells me there is more to the story. For example, I have worked with many overweight people who were raising their grandchildren due to having pregnant teenagers. They loved their beautiful grandchildren, and they wanted to give their daughters/sons a chance to get back on their feet, so they offered to help. They felt guilty taking time to take care of themselves, to have a life. So they didn't and the weight stayed on. They felt depressed.

When they had the courage to look within (by journaling), they would be surprised to see how much anger they felt, how resentful they felt. They didn't like those feelings and stuffed them within, (sometimes with food,) which then developed into a deeper depression.

Let me clarify that I am referring to situational depression that arises when you have excess stress and unresolved feelings. I believe those feelings can be treated, even avoided, provided you are proactive. If you allow it to escalate it can become a complicated problem and even the source of your weight gain. I am not referring to chemical imbalances.

That is a separate issue with a completely different orientation. It is a serious issue that should be treated by a doctor or psychiatrist.

In addition to spiritual faith, the key to happiness and inner peace is all in your attitude. You can overcome almost anything with the right attitude. I am certain that you can create a joyful life even while you are losing weight. With an attitude of gratitude, start by taking back control over your feelings. Rather than seeing life as unfair and getting angry, view life as a gift. One of the gifts of life is that it provides you with a series of wonderful learning experiences.

Jonie's Depression:

Jonie came to see me to lose weight. She was taking care of her aging parents as well as her teenage children. She was a single parent working hard, selflessly and running herself into the ground. I could see that she was under a lot of stress and mentioned this to her several times. She was also being treated for high blood pressure and an autoimmune disorder. Due to her lifestyle, she rarely remembered to take her medication.

One day she came in and was feeling depressed because she wasn't losing any weight. I told her that she needed to make time for health and begin to view this experience with gratitude because it has pushed her so far that she now had to take care of herself instead of everyone else. It fell on deaf ears. I encouraged her to acknowledge her feelings and to ask for help.

Finally I said to her one day, "Do you realize that you might die prematurely because of all of this stress coupled with neglecting your health?" She answered defiantly, "If it is my time, then that is fine with me." I was frustrated and I heard myself respond by saying: "You would do that to your children? Your daughter is planning a family. She's going to want you there, to reassure her, to show her how to do certain things that only a mother can do. What kind of an example of a mother are you going to set – that mothers run themselves into an early grave?"

The expression on her face changed. She said "I never thought about it that way." I said "Remember the first time your baby spiked a fever or had the croupy cough? It was frightening and a young mother wants her mother to assure her that everything will be fine." She had an epiphany and the light switch went on. She immediately took action.

She got help with her parents, started to workout, took her medication, ate healthier and delegated chores. She started taking care of herself, using the reminder of her importance as a parent. She looked back on the experience with gratitude that it helped her to take back control over her health and life. She used it as a reminder to not slip into that old familiar trap again.

When you view life and the events as learning experiences, it is certain to help you to grow and make you a better person. Then acceptance and appreciation follow. For you to successfully create a healthy lifestyle, you will need a healthy outlook on life. I know no better way than to develop an attitude of gratitude. It will help you to put things in perspective.

My prayer for you is that this journey is a peaceful and joyful one. Life is what you make it. Your attitude will determine your results. Give it a try. If you are like most of my clients you will discover a happier you living inside that body you have been criticizing for so long. This you wants to be loved and accepted for who they are right now at this very moment. I hope you entertain this concept and move forward in life with an attitude of gratitude. It is totally up to you and it is your choice.

Here are some suggestions to maintain an attitude of gratitude:

Self-love and acceptance:

I believe the first step is to accept where you are in life and trust that it is teaching you something that will serve you for the rest of you life. People worry that if they accept their body or circumstances, they will not move forward. This is only true if you don't value your health and you are willing to settle for less in life. I find that with acceptance and appreciation comes compassion and a deep desire to improve. Being your best means taking action and improving yourself on a daily basis.

Look at the big picture:

There is a grand plan in life, a purpose bigger than our own selves. Life doesn't revolve around us, and it never will. As much as we would like to think that we are the focus of people and their discussions, we generally are not.

It is our ego that makes us think this, and our ego wants to keep us distracted with petty and self-defeating thoughts. If you could see your whole life and all of the lives that you will impact from your creator's viewpoint, then most of your struggles and experiences would make sense. Because you are in the midst of life, you don't see it, and often focus on the negative feelings. Step back and remind yourself that there is a purpose for everything in life. Be grateful to be part of it.

Count your blessings:

On a daily basis, either record or think about all the reasons you have to be grateful. Think of at least ten reasons. For example: today I am grateful for the time I spent with my daughter, my time to work on this book, the massage I had this morning, the warm breeze while I drank my tea, the new member on my website, my back feeling no pain, my husband kissing me good-bye this morning and smelling so good, and the big hug my son gave me. I play this as a game with my family. I start off with "Today I am grateful for..." and then each person has to come up with something from the day.

Focus on the positive. "Like" attracts "like." That means that you will get more of what you focus on. This will also activate your brain to look for reasons to be grateful. If you have a hard time feeling grateful think of someone you love at the same time, as it will bring up feelings of love and appreciation for you. This may trigger other good memories as well.

When I need a good memory, I think about my children when they were babies and how good it felt to cuddle with them. This settles my mind and brings a sense of peace into my being.

Use challenges to help others:

When you look back on the biggest challenges in life you will see how they have taught you something. One powerful and healing activity is to express gratitude for the challenges in your life. In fact, that is the basic premise and foundation for my entry and success in weight loss coaching. I turned one of my biggest struggles, into a program and tool to help others.

I continue to find this useful and it strengthens me. I actually say, "Thank you, God, for this problem." I use the fact that I gain weight so easily and have to watch my food intake to help others overcome their weight problems as well. I feel blessed to not be able to eat whatever I want. It makes me healthier and it helps me to relate to my clients. When you feel frustrated with one of life's challenges, stop and think of someone you love. Imagine seeing them saying "thank you" to you for sharing your experience with them; imagine that your life has provided someone with hope and inspiration.

Your Assignment:
Practice these techniques. Start to record what you are grateful for in your journal on a daily basis and see how your life changes.

Establishing Your Goals and Outcomes

Goals have been a major reason for my success in life. I grew up being poor. We were on welfare and I remember my mother relying on food stamps to feed us. My mother loved us but had a poverty mindset. The message was "This is the way it is, don't expect more." As I became a teenager, I realized that life offered people around me so much more than I had, I came to believe it was possible for as well. I realized that if I found a job I would be paid for my efforts, and I could in fact have more by being proactive. Very early in life I was recruited into sales, selling cosmetics. I loved wearing makeup and inherited my mother's looks so this was a good match. People wanted to buy what I was using. In sales, goals are crucial to your success. I learned the importance of setting goals. It served me well. I not only used this skill professionally but personally as well.

I cannot tell you how valuable goals are in life. In one study, people who actually wrote down their goals achieved their outcome 95% of the time. People who do not write down their goals achieved their outcome only 5% of the time. This is pretty incredible! If you are serious about being successful in weight management, take a moment to write down your goals.

Let's first clarify the difference between a goal and an outcome. Your outcome is your long-range plan. Where do you want to be 5 years from now? Let's assume you want to be healthy and live to be 100 years old. Your outcome is to live 100 healthy years. Your goal is to maintain a healthy weight to support your ultimate outcome. Goals are steps to help you reach your outcome. You might want to fully consider… "What is your ultimate outcome?" Once you have an answer, ask yourself "What steps do I need to accomplish to reach my outcome?" These will determine your goals.

I invite you to establish your outcome in terms of your health. Your outcome may be to have a healthy body, 25% body fat, low cholesterol, and a healthy heart. Your goals might be, to work out three times a week, cut back on fat, and eat more fresh fruits and vegetables. These goals will lead you to your outcome. Your outcome will take time, your goals will keep you on track. Your goals may differ, but your outcome is always to have a healthy body. Having said that, I also know that goals can consume you.

Goals are intended to motivate you, and keep your feet moving forward. Avoid using goals as another reason to harshly judge yourself. When I was in sales (before I had children), I lived for my goals. I enjoyed sales because of the recognition. My efforts were applauded. Having experienced so much adversity during my life coupled with so little approval, this was a dream come true. What I later discovered was that I was basing my self worth on how much I accomplished rather than who I was. I only allowed myself to feel worthy when I performed well or reached a goal. Once I left sales to stay home with my children, I missed the praise from work.

I found this to be a healing experience because I now had an opportunity to discover who I really was inside and be that person. Just because no one would notice and give me any recognition, it didn't take away from the fact that I was worthy. My epiphany was that if someone else can give me a feeling of worthiness then they could take it away. Why give away my power? I was doing something noble that I loved and I didn't need anyone to validate it to be true.

This was a wonderful lesson for me spiritually. I came to realize that we are all worthy in God's eyes even when we are not accomplishing a goal. Plus I had to ask myself, "Whose goals am I striving for to begin with?"

The goals and outcomes I was shooting for belonged to the younger Rosa who wanted to be number one in sales. The one who really wanted the people who mistreated her and criticized her so harshly to see how wrong they were about her. I was a different person now. I discovered that I was whole, wonderful, and worthy of love even at my darkest hour. My goals and outcomes were completely different now. My main priority was to be the best mother I could be, to raise children who had self-esteem, and felt loved and valued. This was my goal and it was time to claim my power. Why give someone else the power to decide when I will feel like a winner in life and when I do not?

Take back power over your life; you can feel happy whenever you choose. Happiness is within you, not outside of you. Set your goals and outcomes, but decide to be happy throughout the process.

Belinda's Goal:

When Belinda came in, she, like many of my clients weighed over 250 pounds. And at 5'2" she thought that her mission was to lose weight. But her outcome was really to be healthy, have energy, and enjoy her family. If she would have decided that losing weight was her outcome, she might not have gone about it in a healthy manner. But once I explained the difference between outcomes and goals, she realized how achieving overall health was really her outcome.

One goal was to be able to play with her kids without tiring so quickly. She wanted to run around with them, go down a slide, and effortlessly play on the floor lifting her body up without a struggle. Another goal was to weigh under 200 pounds.

As a weight loss coach I've learned many interesting things. One is that when working with people who have never weighed less than 200 pounds in their adult life, this becomes part of their belief system. They unconsciously believe they physically cannot weigh less than 200 pounds. As their weight goes down they start to get nervous. At 210 pounds they are becoming almost apprehensive. They are actually afraid that their body can not do it. They need to change their programming. And most do.

I love it when they finally make this mental breakthrough, because it transforms them. It requires commitment and dedication. When you have a goal that supports your overall outcome you are not going to give up. The goal is only a stepping stone toward an outcome. I asked her to imagine coming into my office and seeing the number 199.5 on my scale. She imagined it with intense feeling daily. I will never forget the day that she stepped on my scale and it read 199 we squealed with delight.

I hugged her and she beamed with pride. The next week when she came in I noticed her fresh makeup (she never wore much before), the week after, and her trendy hair style. At 185 pounds I recall seeing her in an adorable colorful outfit.

She looked beautiful, so much changed within Belinda. This milestone would not be the end of her journey. So many people would go out and celebrate by eating a banana split. Not her, because even though she reached a goal, she was in pursuit of her ultimate outcome. It magnified her motivation.

Here is a simple approach for you to joyfully pursue your outcome:

1. Write down your outcome in your journal.

2. Begin to prepare for its arrival, assuming that if it is for your highest good, God will grant it.

3. Take consistent action in the direction of your outcome. Show yourself that you are serious.

4. Release the attachment to having the outcome; don't let it own you. Thy will be done.

5. Just let go, and trust that if it is in your best interest, it will materialize. Trust in the grand plan in life and have faith.

Here are guidelines in establishing your goals.

- Know what your specific outcome and goals are in detail.

- Be sure they are attainable with your current lifestyle.

- Ask yourself why these goals are important to accomplish.

- Establish a way to measure progress for your goals and outcome.

- Ensure that the goal will support your values and beliefs.

- Give yourself all the time you need to be successful.

- Eliminate obstacles that hold you back, like limiting beliefs.

- Review empowering statements daily, such as beliefs in this book.

Your Assignment

Write down your goals and outcomes. Share them with your team.

The Gift of Time

Changing your diet and making your health a priority takes time. It requires patience, persistence and commitment to do whatever it takes to reach your outcome. Your goal is to lose weight. Your outcome is to live a long healthy, high-quality life. You absolutely deserve both.

If you focus only on the goal of losing weight, you will be discouraged every time you step on the scale and see that you didn't lose a pound. You will be more likely to quit. When you focus on making your health a priority, you are prepared for the journey. Remember, *weight management is a lifestyle not an event.*

An outcome such as living a long life in a healthy, fit body involves wisdom, purpose and time. Remember, with today's medical advances, you will be around for a long time, but it's up to you to determine the quality of your life. The time and energy you put in today will benefit you later. You have a choice: you can live to be 90 years old in a healthy body, walking daily, or you can spend it in a wheelchair in a nursing home.

When I was fourteen, I was diagnosed with scoliosis. I had to have back surgery. I remember that September day I checked into the hospital. I would be there for three weeks. That was the day my doctor and mother told me the truth. I would spend three months at home and the entire school year in a body cast. I cried. I had just started 8th grade and was voted president of the student body. This was a big year for me. I was angry and told the doctor there was nothing wrong with me; I felt healthy.

My doctor said, "Rosa, look at this from the perspective of 20 years from now. This year will be one short episode in your whole life. If you don't do this now, you will regret it later. You will have a host of health problems. Your curve is accelerating quickly and we have to take care of it now. When you are older you will be healthy. You will be glad that you did this. Other people who have this problem and don't have the surgery will have a hunched back and other medical problems. You won't."

As difficult as it was, I looked at that time period of pain and awkwardness as a temporary inconvenience. Today, you would not know I ever had a back problem. My time in that body cast was well-spent. Today, I am very flexible. Many people my age are deteriorating but I am rebuilding. It is all in the way you approach it. I keep reminding myself:

"Am I doing what I need now to live 50 more years?" So I evaluate, and make changes, like adding weight training to my routine. Sometimes I pull a muscle. When that happens, I figure out what I did wrong so that I don't repeat the mistake. I may have to change my workout routine; reduce my weights, rest longer. I am grateful for these learning experiences. I have my whole life to get this right. As long as I am on track 80% of the time, I am successful.

Keep life in perspective. We are often in a hurry because we tell ourselves that our outcome has to be achieved quickly. We fall into the trap of comparing ourselves to others, and then judge ourselves harshly. We exaggerate to ourselves by saying "Jane lost all that weight in six weeks," when it was really eighteen months.

Remember that everything comes with a price. Are you willing to pay the price? I especially am troubled by the messages we are giving our daughters. Look at the cover of any magazine. The message is loud, "The way you look naturally isn't good enough." Sure you can look like a model, provided you have cosmetic surgery, become painfully thin and have your photo altered to eliminate any imperfections! The media is saying that we can't accept women for the way they are. This is outrageous as they are beautiful women who don't need to be "perfected". There is little we can do to change the media, but you can change how you view those messages. You can accept who you are and take the time you need to find the right balance for you to create and maintain a healthy body and lifestyle.

Imagine you are a scientist seeking a cure for a disease. You don't give up when one experiment doesn't work; you keep trying, convinced that the answer is within reach. Well, the answers to your healthy body are within your reach: exercise, healthy eating, and the proper mindset. Take time to create a lifestyle that supports your health. You just have to find the right exercise, the best food plan, and the right attitude for you to stay on track.

It took me an entire year to lose thirty pounds. I would get impatient and think, "Why is this taking so long?" Then I would realize that if I stayed at this pace I would be at my ideal weight next year at this time. This thought would reassure me. That was in 1998 and I haven't regained the weight. I had one year of weight loss and years of my goal! It is worth it.

That is what you want to focus on – a mindset and lifestyle that keeps the weight off and keeps life in perspective.

Your Assignment:

Decide today that you are committed to do what it takes for as long as it takes to reach your outcome. What are some empowering messages you can create and say to yourself that will keep you on track? Here are a couple of beliefs you can begin to say daily.

Thinking Thin Thought:

"I am 100% committed to creating my healthy body."
"I have all of the time I need."

Your Commitment Level

"Until one is committed there is hesitance…That moment one definitely commits oneself, then providence moves too. All sorts of things occur to help one that would otherwise never have occurred. A whole stream of events issues from the decision, raising in one's favor all manner of unforeseen incidents and meetings and material assistance, which no man could have dreamt would come his way." W.N. Murray

This passage had a profound impact on my life. I realized that commitment is essential. You must be 100% committed to your outcome in order to reach it.

When I decided to be 100% committed, my own life changed. My mission became to teach and empower others to create a healthy, happy, and balanced life. I stepped out of my comfort zone in a big way and I took action. I became committed to this mission. I created a comprehensive website, recorded CDs and wrote this book. This took a significant investment of money, as well as time away from my family. I made many mistakes, some of them very expensive, but I was committed to finishing what I started. I even took a full-time job teaching classes to help fund my vision. I stopped focusing on the fear of failure or even the fear of bankruptcy. I focused on how I could help all of the amazing people out there, those people who feel like I once felt.

Here is where the big epiphany came for me: action is secondary. Consistent action is required but it is only secondary. When you are truly committed, you will find the path. Believe me, the path to your outcome is not as important as the commitment to your outcome.

Why do I say this? Because there are thousands of paths to reach your outcome. If you are really committed to your path toward creating a healthy body and lifestyle, then you will achieve that outcome. One goal, or path, will be to lose weight as part of the process of achieving overall health. There are hundreds of paths to accomplish this. You can reduce your calories per day, you can join a program, you can start to exercise, you can read one of the thousands of books about how to lose weight. The actions or paths that you can take are endless to reach your outcome. But unless you are 100% committed, you won't follow through on any of them.

What stops the majority of people in life from reaching their goals and outcomes is a lack of commitment. They say, "I tried everything and it didn't work." Sure it feels true, but it is inaccurate. No one has tried everything. Edison himself tried thousands of experiments until he discovered how to make the light bulb work. Edison was committed to making it work, not looking for excuses.

He knew his outcome was a light bulb and so he kept on his path. Every failed attempt was a learning experience. He has said, "I didn't fail thousands of times, I discovered thousands of ways that didn't work."

Now let me ask you a question and please answer honestly. On a scale from 0% to100%, how committed are you to your outcome – your health? This is your life and your body the only one you are ever going to get. If you really want to make a change you need to be 100% committed. If you are not 100% committed, I understand, as it takes time to get there. Let me ask you another question. How committed are you to figuring this out, to getting yourself to 100%? Sure it will take time, but you have the gift of time. It will require consistent action and I have provided you with guidelines and assignments in this book. You might not get the results that you hoped for but then you can express an attitude of gratitude for what you have learned. Once you change your mindset on this and become 100% committed, your outlook and thought patterns will change in a radical way. Decide to become 100% committed right now! Just do it, this decision will make you unstoppable in all areas of your life.

You might be thinking, "I don't know how to do this. I don't know where to begin." It is simple but not easy. As you know, I am a "thinking thin" kind of woman and I truly believe in everything I am suggesting.

The only way to motivate yourself to be unstoppable – like the quote at the beginning of this chapter – is to decide right now that you are totally and completely committed to doing whatever it takes to reach your goal.

A great example of this kind of commitment is an athlete. Watch any rerun of the Olympics and when the gold medal winner is interviewed the reporter usually asks, "What is going through your mind during the competition?" The answer is often, "I stay focused and think about the crowd cheering for me when I finish, then getting the gold." You will hear this type of answer repeatedly. Why? Because this is what makes them committed to do whatever it takes to succeed. They see the end result and it is with them winning! See yourself winning.

Mentally prepare to do what ever it takes to be unstoppable!

Make a Commitment:

You have to have a strong commitment to success. On a scale of 0-10, zero being no desire and ten meaning you are so excited you can taste it. You have to get yourself committed to 100%, for this is what will drive you. It will be the reason you order the salad, workout when you don't feel like it, and say no when you want to say yes. Ask yourself, "What level am I at now 0-10?" Then ask your self, "Where do I need to be to become unstoppable?" Finally ask the last question, "What will it take for me to get to that level?"

Create a Vision:

To ignite this desire, you must see yourself crossing the finish line. See yourself in an outfit that looks good on you. Plan ahead an event that you want to attend and see yourself dressed up and looking great! If you have children or grandchildren, see yourself playing with them, running and easily keeping up. When I thought about my kids playing I would envision myself racing them down a slide at the playground. Of course I would win and we would do it again I would imagine myself on vacation and I look so good in my bathing suit that my daughter tells me to cover up. Get outrageous and have fun with this.

Take Action:

Be committed to take consistent action and find the right path for you. Nothing happens until you take that first step. This is what makes the difference. If something isn't working, try something different. Using a food journal is the best way to begin.

Write down everything you eat. Track your calories, proteins, carbs, and fats. This will reveal the formula for your body. Then start to move. Have fun, go for a walk, swim, and dance. Just move that sexy body of yours. You must literally flood your brain with positive information on a daily basis. This is how positive habits and learning occur.

Have Faith:

You must believe that you can do this and be grateful that you are on the right track. There is no room for doubt; the minute you lose faith you lose ground. Believe in your ability to be committed and accomplish your outcome. Doubt will weaken you and cause you to focus on losing rather than succeeding.

Surround Yourself with Supportive People

Your state of mind is so important during this process. It is imperative that you surround yourself with positive, supportive people. You will need energy to do all of the things that you need to do to make your health a priority. People will either energize you or drain you. Think of who the positive-energy people are in your life. Notice how you feel when you are around certain people.

If you spend time around people with negative energy, they will distract and discourage you, and after a few minutes you will feel drained.

I'm talking about Complaining Carl at work. He complains about how much work he has and how lazy everyone else is. He can't believe how stupid the company is, and the people they hire have no common sense.

Or how about your friend Martha the Martyr? She has an unmotivated, couch-potato, jobless, adult family member at home who won't help with chores or pay rent. She cooks, cleans, works, and takes care of her parents, while her husband is playing golf. She has endless stories of being unappreciated. When you suggest a solution she responds with, "What's the use?" or "I really don't mind."

You might have a dear friend like Ailing Arthur. You went to high school together and you bump into him frequently around town. You ask him how he is doing and he spends 30 minutes explaining all of his physical problems, the medications he is on, and their side effects.

Maybe you know Whining Wilma, she is convinced that life isn't fair and she has the worst luck of anyone you know. Sweet woman, you wish life would be better for her.

Let's not forget about your brother-in-law, Harsh Harold. He is insensitive and very opinionated. Tough on the outside, soft on the inside, you love him. But he does tend to be overbearing and loves a good "spirited" debate.

And there is Downer Donna. She is well informed on all current events and even has statistics to back up what she says. An innocent comment from you can remind her of a horrific true story she read last week and wants to forewarn you about it.

Don't forget your neighbor, Gossipy Gladys. She has a heart of gold and will do anything for you. You can't help but like her, yet every time you chat she tells you who lost their job, who is getting a divorce, and what happened to Jane's best friend's sister's coworker.

But the real person to watch out for is Sarcastic Sally. She is really funny and makes you laugh. She has a wisecrack and comeback for all kinds of scenarios. She is entertaining and seems to enjoy life at every one else's expense. Sure, her cleverness may seem harmless and entertaining, but notice how you feel after the conversation.

We have all known these people, or, dare I say, even been these people at various times in our lives. In either case, each encounter we have is either energizing or draining. People who dwell on the negative can drag us down.

Ask yourself, "Does this person add to my energy or deplete it?" Be honest with yourself, are you acting like some of these people? We all fall into that trap. If you are, then change what you are saying. Disengage from those types of conversations with yourself and with others. Like attracts like; we are like magnets, unconsciously drawn to what is familiar to us. It is our nature.

I am not suggesting you drop these relationships, just be aware of the effect they may have on you and create some space to re-energize your internal battery and elevate your energy level.

When you are optimistic and peaceful you will spend less time in activities that drain you. They do not interest you or serve a purpose for your life. Good replaces negative, it just happens.

You only have a certain amount of energy on any given day. You are going to need much of it to stay optimistic and focused. There is a lot for you to do in this life, and it will require consistent positive energy and thinking to get you there. Imagine trying to be healthy and Sarcastic Sally is teasing you about how much food you ate. Imagine having the energy to go to the gym and Whining Wilma calls and talks to you. How much energy will you have left to work out? Notice the effects that people, the media and your habitual thoughts have on your energy and attitude.

Thinking Thin Thought:
"I deserve to be surrounded by loving, supportive & nurturing people."

A Community of Choice

Surround yourself with positive, supportive, upbeat people. Make a list of people who support, energize, and inspire you. You will want to include friends whose lives don't revolve around food. Seek out fitness friends who like to be active and engage in physical activities. List some optimistic friends who really believe life is awesome and genuinely enjoy the process of everyday living. I also recommend adding spiritual friends, who are motivated by a purpose greater than themselves.

I call this a community of choice. You can't pick your family but you can pick your friends. Begin to create a community of wonderful, uplifting, and supportive people. This will increase the quality of your life and help you to reprogram your mind for success in all your goals and outcomes. In sales they told us, we become like the five people we spend the most time with. Who are you spending time with? Do you want to be like them? You can still be kind and compassionate to everyone, just broaden your circle to include supportive people.

Your Assignment

Create a community of choice.

1. Make a list of supportive, encouraging & energizing people in your life.

2. What are the qualities about these people that you like?

3. Where else can you meet more people like this?

4. Make a decision to spend time with supportive people.

5. Meet with your team to follow this program.

6. Visit MindOverPlatter.com's chat room to talk to like-minded individuals: http://www.mindoverplatter.com/chat/chat/index.php3

Treat Yourself with TLC

In addition to others draining you with negativity, are you hard on yourself? Do you set yourself up to feel bad even when you have made progress? Do you tend to encourage everyone else, yet not give yourself credit for all of your efforts? If you are answering "yes" to the above questions, then it is time to treat yourself with tender loving care.

Many people who struggle with their weight tend to have caretaker personality styles. This in part is due to an internal rule that tells them to be nice. This same rule tells them if they're not nice to everyone all of the time then they are being selfish. What an ugly word, selfish. If we only allow ourselves to feel good when we are taking care of others or doing something that benefits others, then we might be classic caretakers.

Caretakers want to be seen as loving, kind, and considerate. The worst thing for a caretaker personality is the fear of being seen as selfish. Are you a caretaker? If you are, then you have mastered the ability of pleasing everyone else while putting yourself last. You are probably the first person people call when they need a favor. You know exactly what to say when someone has had a bad day to comfort them. You are a talented communicator and make people feel special and valuable. This is one of your gifts; few people have it my friend, but you do.

I was a caretaker, for my little sisters and brother, from age five and up and then, for my mother. When I finally hit maximum capacity: the energy and pain involved in being a caretaker became greater than the pain involved in forcing myself to be selfish and take care of me.

It is a blessing to have the gift of mercy, compassion and caretaking. For me it is a spiritual gift that could serve well when people need counseling, guidance, or companionship.

There are two concerns that I have with this gift:

1. People may easily take advantage of your good heart.

2. You are not saving any of that great advice, compassion, and encouragement for yourself.

When you do make a mistake, you are angry with yourself and criticize yourself harshly. You would never treat a friend the way you treat yourself. It is time to take care of yourself. You definitely deserve it. A word of caution: you never really overcome having a caretaker personality. It is always there and can sneak up on you again if you aren't paying attention.

When God created you to be so kind, it is my belief that it was never the intention to sacrifice your health and mental well-being. Everyone needs a balance. Stop beating yourself up and start to speak kindly to yourself. Decide that you have overlooked a lifelong friend who you have neglected for years – you! Notice all of the wonderful things you do for others and extend that kindness to yourself. Come from a place of gratitude. It will transform your self-image.

Your Assignment:

Time for TLC

Each morning as you are getting ready for your day, be mindful of your body. Begin while showering. Take the time to use lotion or sweet almond oil and rub it into your skin, express gratitude and love to your body, feel peaceful. Try it. The worst thing that will happen is that you will be clean, soft, and at peace.

The Mind/Body Connection and Weight Management

"All that we are is the result of what we have thought. The mind is everything. What we think, we become." - Maharishi Mahesh Yogi

It is important to invite the power of your brilliant mind to help you lose weight and be healthy. If your head is in the wrong place, whatever you try won't work. You can seem to be doing everything right but make little progress.

When your head is in the right place, everything you do will seem to work. If you are serious about losing weight, which I know you are, then you will want to enlist the support of your mind. It will be the difference between a lifelong battle or a natural way of being.

Your thoughts are powerful and they have a dramatic effect on your body. If you don't believe that the mind and body are affecting each other, try this simple exercise: close your eyes and pretend that there is a big juicy yellow lemon sitting on your kitchen counter. Then imagine you take out a cutting board and your favorite paring knife and cut that lemon in half! Imagine the juice is squirting out all over your fingers. Then imagine you cut the half lemon into quarters. Now take one of those quarter hunks of juicy ripe lemon and bring it towards your mouth. Pretend that you are really biting into it, taste the cold tangy sour juice, feel the texture of the pulp in your mouth, the smooth but course rind in your fingers. Pretend you can smell the lemon's citrus fresh scent. And notice how much saliva forms in your mouth as you do this.

Now you know there is no lemon; you know that you did not touch, smell, or taste a lemon. Yet, you formed saliva and may have even puckered from the thought. The reason is that the mind and body are connected. The mind has a thought which signals emotions, which then causes a physical response. This is also known as a psychosomatic response.

To help you understand this process better let's explore the mind.

You have a conscious mind and a subconscious mind

The conscious mind is logical and analytical. It evaluates and reasons, continually comparing information and cross-referencing it with what is taking place. The conscious mind is suspicious by nature. Its primary function is to protect you and keep you safe. It is thinking, "What is happening right now and what does this mean to me?" It then goes to its many references: past experiences, memories, future expectations, and intellect, to determine how to respond.

Let's look at the example of believing you are good in math. Your conscious mind will approach this analytically, by cross-referencing data: you always received an "A" in math both in high school and college, you balance your checkbook with little effort, and you are often the person who figures out what everyone owes when you go out to dinner.

So, your conscious mind will respond with, "Yes, all of the evidence points to the fact that I am good in math." It needs a level of logic to agree and reinforce what you believe. Making a change on the conscious level requires time, consistent repetition, reinforcement and willpower – until your conscious mind is satisfied with the data, in which case it grabs the belief and holds on tightly.

The subconscious mind is creative and free-flowing. It is not evaluating, it is trusting and cooperative. It does not judge you or your beliefs. It is here to serve you always. It is vital for your survival. Your subconscious mind ensures that your breathing is regulated, your heart is beating, and it is also in charge of your organs and glands. It takes care of you, even when you are not aware of it. The subconscious mind is a very important and powerful part of your mind. Anything that you do while on autopilot is done by your subconscious mind. Think about driving; how many times have you thought, "Did I just pass my exit? I don't remember driving this long." Because of the efficiency of your unconscious mind, you can do multiple vital tasks simultaneously and successfully.

Your subconscious mind's main function is to keep you alive. It is thinking, "What can I do for you?" When you have a thought such as, "I am good in math" it responds with "Okay, your thought is my command!"

It needs no proof, it doesn't know the difference between reality and the imagined. If you think it is true, then to the subconscious mind it is true.

All of your habits and beliefs are stored in your subconscious mind as well. If I asked you to tie your shoes, you would just do it without thinking. That is because it is stored in the subconscious mind as a habit after having done it hundreds of times. Your beliefs are a result of programming, years of hearing certain messages, and thus believing them. This is how your self-image is created, how you see yourself unconsciously. We call that your self-image. Many of my clients have never weighed less than 200 pounds in their adult lives. Their self-image involves believing that they will never weigh less than 200 pounds. The subconscious mind obeys the command and responds with, "Okay, you will never weigh less than 200 pounds. Anything else I can do for you?"

Your self-image, habits, and beliefs are the result of years of conditioning and repetition. You may have thought consciously, "I can't lose weight." The conscious mind says, "Maybe yes, maybe no, that remains to be seen. Your mother is overweight and genetics do play a role, if I exercise and eat a balanced diet I could probably lose weight. It worked for Aunt Maple and she was really overweight."

Your subconscious mind responds with, "Okay, I will lose weight if I exercise." Then your conscious mind continues, "I hate exercise. Remember the last time I paid all of that money to join a gym. I only went a few times then pulled a muscle; with my luck I'll do that again."

Your subconscious mind responds with, "Okay, exercise is expensive and I will only get hurt. I will store this information right away, anything else I can do for you?" So when you go begin an exercise program the conscious mind says, "I don't know if this is going to work, but I will give it a try. I hope I don't hurt myself." Your subconscious mind says, "EXERCISE? This is in conflict with my programming. I hate exercise, gyms are too expensive and I will only pull a muscle and hurt myself.". So you (unconsciously) pick a workout that pushes you and is not the best match for your fitness level. What happens? You pull a muscle and hurt yourself. Your conscious mind says "I knew it!" The subconscious mind will never disappoint you. To make a lifelong change you will want the subconscious mind on board.

Think of the conscious and subconscious mind as a computer. The conscious mind is like your computer screen. What you see displayed is based on what you have asked for, which files you are focused on at the moment. However, it is only a fraction of what is available within the system. It can cross-reference information and do difficult tasks. When you ask the right way, it will do amazing things for you.

What determines this is your skill level in knowing which sequence of keys to push to create a command that will retrieve the results you are looking for. The conscious mind is the same way. Your results are based on where you focus your attention and knowing what your destination is.

The subconscious mind is like the database. It doesn't judge or evaluate what it is asked to do. It simply serves. It is not navigating or creating a game plan, it just follows the path it is told to. It can store millions of files in your database and call them up within a fraction of a second; all you need to do is ask. Those files will be stored permanently unless you decide to edit, replace, or delete them. The subconscious mind wants to please you; it is here to serve you. The key is in the programming, as the saying goes, "Garbage in, garbage out." You will learn how to reprogram your mind to support your goals.

So, in essence, by focusing your results on health and fitness your subconscious mind will supply your conscious mind with everything it needs to accomplish your goal. They need to work together. In order for you to successfully reprogram your mind from self-limiting thoughts to empowering thoughts you have to bypass the filter between the two, which is known as critical filter. In the computer world it would be known as the firewall, it that scans every single file before it allows it to be stored in the database.

This filter (firewall) is based on your criteria – your values, beliefs, likes, and dislikes. It is in place to protect you and has developed over time. For example let's assume you resent sales calls during dinner hour. Now imagine it is 6:30 pm. You are enjoying dinner and the phone rings. The person calling asks for the head of the household, and you might suspect it is an unsolicited telemarketing call. Your critical filter will be high because you don't want what the caller is offering. You will feel suspicious and very resistant to having a conversation with them. Therefore, the suggestions the person is making will not be successful because your critical filter is on high alert.

Let's assume a few minutes later the phone rings again and your critical filter is still on high alert but this time the voice is someone whom you know and love. Your critical filter will reduce dramatically and your response will immediately change.

Information passes from the conscious mind to the subconscious mind quickly and easily when your critical filter is low. An effective way to lower your critical filter is by learning how to relax, easing your mind, and letting it settle peacefully. We will discuss ways to do this later in the book.

"Imagination is more powerful than knowledge." – Albert Einstein

Once you have made a conscious decision to be naturally thin, you will need to enlist the subconscious mind's support. This will ensure your success. What is the best way to gain this support? Your imagination, as it easily bypasses your critical filter. This is because your imagination is automatically granted access to your subconscious mind. It is simply programmed that way. The subconscious mind responds to images, emotions, and stories. The key to creating what you want is to use your imagination. Nothing has ever been created without the use of the imagination; it is more powerful than willpower.

Whenever you position willpower against imagination, willpower will always lose. Let's compare a chronic dieter to a naturally thin person who both see a piece of chocolate cake. The chronic dieter's willpower will only last for a few minutes, and then imagination kicks in. They begin to fantasize about how luscious the chocolate frosting looks. They imagine the texture of the cake in their mouth and the richness of the frosting, followed by a sip of perfectly brewed coffee. They feel hungry and crave the cake. Need I continue? Are you salivating? I know I am. How can you resist? Imagination wins and willpower loses, you eat the cake.

This is exactly what we do, use our imagination to stay fat and crave food. Now the naturally thin person sees the cake and stops there. She imagines stepping on the scale and it is up five pounds, she sees her jeans not zipping up, she thinks about the workout this morning and says "No way, I work too hard to stay this size." She applies willpower with imagination. When you have imagination and willpower on the same team, you win. This combination is crucial in creating a true change.

As your virtual weight loss coach, I want you to enlist your powerful subconscious mind by activating your imagination! Let your mind get curious about what it would be like to live in a healthy and fit body. What types of clothes will you wear? How will you carry your body? Where will you go in your amazing body? This is fun and easy. Just allow yourself to pretend.

Remember when you were a child and you would pretend? You know how to do this, you were born doing this. It is a proven fact that your subconscious mind doesn't have the ability to distinguish between reality and imagination. It will believe what you tell it and start to look for a way to manifest it. Stop telling it that you are overweight and unworthy and tell it to get curious about being healthy, fit, attractive – sexy! Just do it, see it, hear it, feel it, sense it, smell it. Do whatever works for you. You don't have to see pictures to use your imagination. Use the same part of your mind that enjoys reading a good book. Imagine yourself healthy; imagine the "You" that you have always wanted to be.

What You Focus on Emerges

"When the mind settles on the mountain, it becomes the mountain."

Thich Nhat Hanh

Your brain is complex and amazing, the mind is beyond the brain. Like the relationship between your body and your soul. A soul occupies the body but never dies, it is an energy that cannot be measured or proven by scientific standards. But most people will agree we have a soul, it is what makes us who we are. The body is an incredible shell that the soul uses for its purpose. I believe God ordains each of us with unique gifts and talents and wants us to use them to serve the world, but that is an entirely different topic for now.

The mind is like your brain's soul, it is everywhere scanning, sorting and searching for what is in your internal programming. If you are following God's original program then you are on the right path. If however, you have been programmed by your family, the media, politics, negative religion or friends, your path may not be the one you chose or even in your best interest.

Within your mind there is a conscious mind (logical and analytical) and your subconscious mind (creative and free flowing). There are literally millions of things your mind could focus on at any given moment. There are trees, the sun, colors, comments people make, the radio, background noise, your thoughts, etc.

What you focus on is based on the Reticulating Activating System (RAS), the part of your brain that unconsciously scans your surroundings for what you are looking for. Once it finds the item you are looking for, it alerts your conscious mind. Let me repeat this because it is true, your brain unconsciously scans your surroundings for what you are looking for. Once it finds it, your conscious mind is alerted. RAS is your mind's antenna, constantly searching for the "frequency" that you are tuned into. My husband loves NASCAR and when we travel he can spot a store that has a car he has been looking for with an uncanny ability. It is amazing. How is this possible? Well your conscious mind can pay attention to as many as 9 things at any moment. Your subconscious mind is aware of millions of things simultaneously.

For example if you were standing at a store and a person grabbed money from the cash register and ran to their car and drove away. You would consciously remember their sex, height, body frame, skin color, hair color, eye color, clothing, noticeable birthmarks, and perhaps the color and the type of car.

Your subconscious mind has observed far more with extraordinary detail. For example you unconsciously witnessed the persons: height, body frame, skin color, markings like tattoos and beauty marks, the type of clothes they were wearing like their shoes, name brands, hair color, eye color, color and make of car, the license plate number and if you saw their drivers license you could recall the ID number as well. This has been proven in the field of forensic hypnosis, where hypnosis is used to help witnesses recall details of a crime with incredible accuracy. I have personally recalled memories while in hypnosis that I was too young to remember, but my mother has confirmed to be true. The mind observes EVERY THING. What you want is out there, are you tuning into it?

Now how does your brain go from millions of observations to nine? The filter in your brain and nervous system is "wired" to process a certain amount of information or else you will feel overwhelmed. Because there is too much occurring in the world the mind has to decide what is most relevant to you and will support your outcome. It will bring to awareness what resonates with what you decided is important for you. This will literally become a self-fulfilling prophecy. It is my belief that nothing will manifest in your outside world unless you make it real in your inside world.

Years ago I went to a holiday party and a friend was wearing an attractive outfit. She had black velvet pants a white silk blouse and a red velvet vest. She was much younger than me and much thinner. She looked great, I complemented her and secretly wished I could look that good. Months later I was mall walking and noticed a big sale. Guess what they had? Not only black velvet pants but a red vest as well. The only size left was too small for me, but I bought it. I couldn't wear it for a couple of years. But one day it fit! I felt great in it. Now I am currently wearing a size smaller. Don't limit yourself, use your imagination, it is fun and relaxing.

Breaking Bad Habits 101

There is nothing mystical about how habits are formed. Habits are simply conditioned responses and/or behaviors. They are the product of conditioning as the result of repetition. You can label almost any action as a habit. Tying your shoes, signing your name, starting your car, can all be considered habits. You probably don't mind those types of habits because the outcome is productive.

When we notice patterns in life that we don't like, they are often the result of bad habits. Once we recognize a bad habit, we are empowered to change it. Habits in themselves are not good or bad they are just conditioned responses. They don't exist because you have deep psychological problems, they have simply occurred because you have done something repeatedly until it crossed the conscious / subconscious critical filter and is now rooted in the subconscious mind. The best way to break a bad habit is to replace it with a positive one. There are two types of habits, empty habits and habits that provide secondary gain.

The difference between an empty habit and secondary gain: An empty habit is the one described above, it is only in your life because you have conditioned it without a reason. When my stepson worked at a pizzeria, he would often bring my husband and I a pizza or a calzone at night after work. Now I wasn't hungry, but it smelled good and I am Italian and love that kind of food. So I would pull up a chair, my kids would come running downstairs, and we would have a little party. It was fun. I enjoyed seeing my family, we were all laughing together. My husband was thrilled to see his son. My kids loved seeing their big brother. It's a good memory for me. It didn't take long, only about a week and I started to crave pizza at night, I wasn't hungry, it was an empty habit. I conditioned eating food at night. All I needed to do was not eat at night and condition that instead, until it became my new habit. Empty habits respond very well to self-hypnosis and all the techniques that I am teaching you in this book.

Now if there is a purpose behind the habit then we call that secondary gain. For me there actually was a purpose for this habit. Let's look deeper into this habit and explore secondary gain.

Secondary gain is an indication that something is going on under the surface. Maybe emotionally, it serves you in some way, which is why you hold on to it. You must address secondary gain if it is not an empty habit. When I realized I conditioned eating at night, I also had to identify any secondary gain, asking myself what the purpose of this habit would be. I quickly realized that I liked seeing my stepson, and him bringing me food meant he loved me (very true in an Italian family). I also liked my kids getting excited to stay up late and we ate and talked, it was fun. My husband was happy, the kids were happy, and I felt connected to my family.

Since family is such a high value for me, it made sense that this was a habit I could easily keep. I instead decided to meet my need of time with my family and sit at the table, but I would choose to sip tea instead of eat. I didn't take away the purpose for the habit just the eating at night part.

For a habit to change, you have to satisfy the underlying need that is being met. This is what is motivating you to take action. You must have a strong "why". People won't change without a reason, therefore, you will want to identify the reason this habit needs to change. Sometimes this alone facilitates the change in itself. So find a solid, strong reason why you want to create a powerful new habit.

John's Habit:

I once worked with a playful client named John. He loved chocolate ice cream and said he wanted to give up that habit permanently. He would joke with me about his love of chocolate especially chocolate ice cream and his boring home life. Weeks went by with little success. He was still eating a bowl of chocolate ice cream every night. I tried everything to help him and he would smile at me and tell me about his latest chocolate ice cream flavor that he found and how wonderful it was. I finally said "John you really don't want to give up your chocolate ice cream do you?" He burst into laughter and said, "No I don't want to give up my chocolate ice cream, I love it." I said then "Why are you here?" He replied, "Because I wanted to see if this would work." I explained to John that he was experiencing secondary gain, and my guess was that ice cream was replacing a desire for companionship. He agreed.

Now he had a choice to address the real issue, which was his loneliness, or continue to eat chocolate ice cream to comfort him. He needed to find a strong enough reason to give it up. It wasn't a simple solution for him, his weight was within a healthy range and he didn't abuse chocolate, he had to decide to change and know why he wanted to do it.

Your Assignment

Identify your habits. Keeping a diary and a food journal will assist you in breaking unhealthy habits and replacing them with healthier habits. I encourage you to use them daily for at least 21 days. An old trick to break a bad habit is to wear a rubber band around your wrist, each time you engage in the old habit, give the band a gentle pull and let it lightly snap against your wrist. This will help you to identify discomfort with the old bad habit. I call it the "snap out of it" technique. But be gentle, I only want you to do it as a reminder to change not a punishment.

This will give you enough information to know where you need to put your focus. You might notice that a certain time of day or a particular meal presents a special challenge for you. Or maybe certain times with friends and family. We will discuss this further in the Food Triggers chapter. Those are your opportunities to apply the steps to changing a habit.

How a habit is formed

1. Action is taken (You eat ice cream at night.)
2. You receive feedback (The ice cream tastes good and provides comfort.)
3. You consistently repeat the action (You continue to eat ice cream at night.)
4. You consistently receive feedback (The ice cream is comforting.)
5. This pattern crosses the conscious/subconscious critical filter until it is rooted in the subconscious mind.
6. A habit is born.

Steps to Changing a Habit

1. Define the habit that you don't want.
2. Ask yourself what is the purpose of the habit.
3. Decide what you want instead - be specific.
4. Be sure to meet the underlying need if there is one.
5. Identify why you want to change this habit: what will it give you?
6. Break the pattern (which is the habit in action).
7. Replace the negative habit with the desired outcome.
8. Condition this consistently for at least 21 days.
9. Reinforce it daily until you effortlessly experience your desired outcome, instead of the old outcome.

How to Create an Action Plan:

Create an action plan to change a habit:

1. What is the habit you don't want?

2. What is the purpose of this habit?

3. What is another way to meet this need?

4. What habit would better serve you instead?

5. What action can you take to interrupt this habit?

6. Why is it important for you to change this habit?

Self Discipline

Have you lost weight only to gain it back? Do you wonder why you will do what works such as exercising and eating healthy only to stop even though you are making progress and seeing results? What causes this?

Is it a lack of motivation? Low self-esteem? A deep-seeded psychological reason rooted in your childhood? After working with thousands of clients I have come to believe it is due to a lack of self-discipline. The key difference between a person who works out daily and one who won't (provided they are the same age, weight, and health), is self-discipline. One person is willing to do something they don't feel like, while the other rationalizes doing it later or not at all.

I did some research studying the science of self-discipline. I thought I would just follow a step-by-step program, but there are few books written about it. There are many written about overcoming procrastination, but don't you need self-discipline to do that? I would say absolutely you do.

I have been pouring over what little I have found and have come up with an outline for you to follow to increase your level of self-discipline. It is very simplistic, but what I find in life is the best-kept secrets often are.

Self-discipline by my definition means, managing one's behavior for the sake of improvement. I think of it as delaying gratification. It doesn't mean saying "no", or denial, it only means postponing. It is a wise choice you make that will strengthen you mentally, physically and emotionally.

The pre-steps to self-discipline:

1. Know what it is that you want.
2. Know why you want it. If you don't know why it is important for you then you will lose the motivation for it.
3. Be sure it is congruent with your values. If you are in conflict, you won't follow through.
4. Have a plan in place to accomplish your goal. Document your progress along the way.

Now here is how you actually develop self-discipline:

1. Practice delaying gratification, for example, if you love to read the newspaper in the morning, postpone it until after you workout. It will motivate you and will help you to strengthen your self-control.

2. Say no to yourself with the sole purpose of strengthening self-control. An example of this is when you want to finish the food on your plate, instead think "I will feel better if I don't" then walk away. Notice how proud you will feel of yourself.

3. Do something that you don't feel like doing such as taking the stairs vs. the elevator, or sending the kids upstairs for you.

4. Be consistent, you must condition your mind to become disciplined, repetition is very important. The brain learns from spatial repetition.

5. Visualize yourself having accomplished what you want. It will motivate you and keep you on track.

6. Never give up, be willing to do what it takes to reach your goal. Persistence is vital for your success.

7. Celebrate your success, feel the joy of accomplishment.

8. Establish a ritual that celebrates your success. My kids and I make a fist and yell "yes". If we go on a ride at the amusement park, the minute we get off and feel the adrenaline rush we say "yes" with our fist. It stores this powerful memory in the body.

This is also known as a trigger. Think about a song you loved in high school, it brings back all kinds of memories. You can establish a trigger to help you develop discipline just as simply.

Establish a Ritual of Success

People who seem to be disciplined also seem to follow a schedule, a routine that when followed keeps them on track. This can also be called a ritual.

A ritual is a pattern that is repeated on a regular basis, like brushing your teeth prior to going to bed. The brain loves patterns and rituals. We have all heard that babies like schedules and kids respond well to routine. I ran a daycare for nearly 10 years and found that to be absolutely true. They not only liked it they thrived while on it. We like to feel a sense of control over our lives, it empowers us.

I refer to it as a ritual, because I choose to partake in it and I don't like the word routine, it sounds too boring for my mind. But ritual means I am disciplined and I value this practice. We have rituals for everything, getting ready in the morning, going to bed, paying the bills, you name it. Think about something you do well and identify the ritual that you use to be successful.

My ritual for inner peace is praying and meditating daily when I wake up and before bed. It reminds my brain and nervous system, "It is time to relax and feel peaceful." As long as I practice this ritual daily no matter what happens in between, I have a good day.

What part of your life is most out of balance? Your health, spirituality, family, self-esteem, choose what first popped into your head. Create a ritual for that one area of your life and start today. For example if you thought, "My eating is out of control- I am eating too much sugar." Then establish a ritual to overcome that successfully. Maybe you will begin by having a protein drink in the morning to stabilize your blood sugar. You may realize that you crave something sweet at 3:00pm, instead have a cup of sugar free cocoa instead. This simple act will soon become a habit and replace the unhealthy one. You are replacing an unhealthy ritual with a healthy one.

If you don't know where to begin, then ask someone who has mastered what you want. They have healthy rituals for success, all you need to do is duplicate it and you will get the same results.

Another option is to think of a time you felt successful in this area and ask yourself what you did to achieve results. You will discover your ritual and all you need to do is duplicate the same steps and self talk.

Your Assignment:

- ☐ Identify one area of your life that you need to implement a ritual for success.

- ☐ Discuss this with your team; it may help them with their ritual as well.

- ☐ Support each other in establishing rituals for success.

Leverage: Why Bother?

Leverage relates to what is driving you to finally go through with something.

If you are within 10 pounds of your ideal weight, your clothes fit fine, and your doctor said your numbers are ideal then you won't have much leverage to change your eating habits. Yet let's assume you develop an allergy to wheat and you break out in hives every time you eat a food with wheat in it, now you have leverage. The leverage is what is bringing you to the point of action. People often don't follow through until they have leverage. And it is very often the painful kind. You have gained too much weight, your clothes don't fit, someone comments on your weight and you feel a sense of urgency to change. You are motivated and determined, which will ignite your discipline.

You must have leverage or you won't follow this program to completion. How do you get leverage? You can gain leverage from either pain or pleasure. Pain is what we just described: unpleasant motivation. Pleasure is hope and happiness, it enriches your life. People either exercise to avoid the pain of being overweight or to seek the pleasure of how good they will look and feel, or a combination of both.

The important point here is to find your internal leverage. What leverage do you need to motivate you? Do you want to watch your kids grow up? Do you want to wear a certain size clothing? Are you worried about your health? Are you more motivated by pain: the fear of something bad happening? Or pleasure: the desire to experience something fun and enjoyable? You need leverage and you need to use your primary driver (pain or pleasure), to propel you or this will only be a phase in your life.

Your Assignment:

What is your leverage in this process?

Discuss it with your weight loss support team.

Distractions

Distractions drain you of precious energy. These are things that take up space in your mind. Unpaid bills, overdue library books, needing to put gas in your car, the birthday card you forgot to mail. These distractions will rob you of your time and, if your not careful, your life.

Now, I think I know people pretty well, especially overweight people. They are the most loving, caring, and giving people on the planet. And they will allow themselves to serve everyone until they can't stand up and finally fall over. I have seen it for years. They simply don't have the energy for themselves because there is too much to do for everyone else.

To lose weight and keep it off you will need to make your health a priority, my dear friend. And to make your health a priority you will need energy. I am saying this from my own lifetime of experience – not only as a weight loss coach, but also as a mother, wife, daughter and sister. You must eliminate or drastically reduce unnecessary distractions in your life. It is time to make time for you!

You need time… time to plan your meals, time to buy groceries, time to prepare your meals and time to exercise. You will also need time to relax and have some fun. If you are going to change your life self-care is an absolute must in my book. As your virtual weight loss coach, I hope it soon becomes a page in yours, as well.

If you haven't accomplished what you have hoped in your life, it may likely be because your goals are not a priority for you. Have you placed everyone else's needs above your own? Are allowing these distractions keeping you from your goal? If so, stop making up excuses for not honoring yourself enough to take care of you. It is your choice. It is not healthy to put your health and well-being on hold for everything and everyone else. It is time to reduce, eliminate or (here comes my favorite word) delegate. Oh how I love to delegate!

Delegate the distractions in your life. Who says they are your responsibility, anyway. It is only your ego that tells you that you have to do it or it will be "wrong." You are not in charge of doing everything and you are not in charge of doing it all perfectly right either. There is no such thing as perfect; it is an illusion. Start delegating today.

Distractions (to name a few), include talking on the phone, worrying about others, letting things pile up until you feel overwhelmed, co-dependent behavior, over-committing, saying "yes" when you mean "no," and any form of gossip. The list goes on and on and on.

I have been there and done that. I was raised by alcoholics and then married to an alcoholic for years. I felt like I was born to take care of everyone but myself. And I must admit I was pretty good at it. I ran the household, managed everyone's schedules, ran a business, painted, decorated, crafted, ran my daughters Brownie troop, and was Vice President of my PTA group. My health was marginal at the time. I was only 28 years old and exhausted.

Thank God for good counselors and my small spiritual group, because I finally used that solid backbone of mine and started to say "No" to everyone else and "Yes" to me. I will share a secret with you… eventually the guilt passes! In fact, at some point you don't even remember to feel guilty – oh what joy that is!

I have a few rules, I will share with you:

➢ I won't do something for someone else that they can do for themselves.

➢ I am willing to help when someone is in crisis, but I get to decide what constitutes a crisis. * I love that saying: "Lack of planning on your part does not constitute a crisis on my part."

➢ I am not queen bee anymore and I don't have the responsibility or even the right to decide what everyone is supposed to do.

➢ I trust in a grand plan: everyone has the experiences they have for a reason.

➢ I will not interfere with someone's choice to learn from their mistakes.

If you're shocked that I'm suggesting these seemingly cold and selfish things, that's okay by me. We are talking change here; change in the way we do things. If you are going to change, you may have to consider applying some of these rules to your own life.

I have come a long way, and I personally know how liberating this can be. I share my personal story with you for a reason. I don't want you to feel bad for me. I want you to know that if I could do it, you can do it!

I won't say to you, "That's okay, you had it rough, and this positive way of thinking and changing your mindset won't work for you." No way! Instead I will say "Listen, friend, this is what I had to say to myself to overcome my own negative programming. Now go ahead and give it all you got. Because I have great news for you, it really works!"

To be successful with this program you will need to make time for it, which means eliminating or drastically reducing your distractions. See the example given below.

Identify your distractions. The ones that once you address, you will be able to relax. Don't put these off any longer, delegate them or just take care of them and notice the difference in your peace of mind and attitude. Then notice the energy you have for YOUR life.

Where are your distractions?

What I want more of in my life? Which distractions are holding me back?

What I want more of in my life?	Which distractions are holding me back?
Time to exercise	*I watch television and lose track of time.*
Quiet time	*I am on the phone comforting a friend.*
Not feel so rushed in my life	*I wait to the last minute to leave.*
Romance	*Lack of planning alone time with mate.*

Your Assignment: Identify your distractions

What I want more of in my life? Which distractions are holding me back?

Emotional Eating, Trance or Physical Hunger

We are looking at so many aspects of our mind. Let's talk about some reasons why we overeat including: emotional, being in a trance, or physical hunger.

Emotional hunger will trace back to stress, anxiety, as well as many feelings, both good and bad. I call these good and bad messages "the committee." When you are listening to the negative messages on the "committee," you are not listening to your heart.

Being in a trance is eating when you are conditioned to eat. It is also known as an empty habit. You have done this so many times that you aren't even aware of what just happened. It's like eating popcorn during a movie. You are not being fully present.

Physical hunger is not paying attention to your stomach or its signals. This leads you to not being aware of when you are hungry or even full. You are not listening to your body. For example if you are engrossed in a project and your stomach begins to growl, and you are feeling light headed, you look at the clock and realized that it has been 6 hours since you last ate. This is true physical hunger, except you waited until you were too hungry and weren't taking care of your body's needs.

When you fall into these habits and patterns it usually leads to overeating, and you lose sight of the fact that you are an amazing and resourceful person. You forget how beautiful and gifted you truly are. Falling into that trap can easily discourage you.

Do not allow yourself to become distracted from your real purpose of creating a happier and healthier life. Remember that you are more than your emotions, more than your habits and more than your body. As author, Dr. Wayne Dyer says, "You are not your body, you have a body. You are not your thoughts, you have thoughts. And you are not your feelings, you have feelings. You are a spiritual being having a human experience."

Know this is true for you. You are capable of a great human experience. Imagine yourself fit and healthy, and you will let go of the excess weight. You will be drawn toward the "you" that you have lost touch with. This is the true you. It begins with listening to your heart, listening to your body and listening to empowering messages from your mind.

This honors your inner truth, your spirit. The true you is so beautiful, so magnificent and yes, divinely guided. Pause for a moment to recognize this is possible. As you do this you may even begin to notice that you crave to experience this peaceful authentic comfort more often than the false comfort of overeating.

Thinking Thin Thought:

"I am committed to me, I will do whatever it takes to honor my true self. I am worth it."

Emotional Eating

The best way to deal with emotional eating is to stop before you begin. Start by noticing your feelings. Then take a deep breath, hold it in for a moment, and slowly exhale. This will help you to relax. Ask yourself, "Am I truly physically hungry right now?" If you are unsure, have a glass of water. Often, your body is thirsty. The brain uses the same signal for thirst as hunger so check out thirst first.

If you are hungry, begin to rate your physical hunger. One is famished, ten is stuffed. Start a habit of eating when you experience a physical rating of a 2, then eat a small balanced portion of food. Once you are satisfied (which is a rating of 5), simply stop and take a deep breath. If you are still feeling the urge to eat, and then ask yourself, "What am I feeling right now?" You might notice you are feeling lonely which could mean you have an unmet need identifying itself. You could be feeling bored, having some "down time" is good for you but you labeled it "boredom".

When these emotions surface, don't judge them, observe them. Feelings that surface do not mean they are accurate. You may find it useful to write in a journal when experiencing these emotions. You will feel better by acknowledging how you feel, notice how fast they lose their power.

It may have been a long time since you have addressed these emotions. Trust that emotions are fickle and they come and go. Feel them and release them with love.

Sometimes the food is filling a need that you haven't met in another way. If this is true for you, find out what this need is and find another way to meet this need without the use of food. Meditation is an excellent way of allowing another solution to surface. Believe in your ability to seek a resourceful alternative like: calling a friend, doing something creative, taking a class, and even finding a fun way to move your body.

Your Assignment:

Use the checklists provided to raise your awareness about when you eat.

Emotional Eating Checklist

Awareness is vital to changing a pattern, list below what you do when these emotions are present. If you do eat, list which foods you choose.

Nervous

Happy

Sad

Bored

Frustrated

Lonely

Fearful

Angry

Joyful

Anxious

Overwhelmed

Tired

Thinking Thin Thought:

"I release the need to comfort myself with food. Food is not a source of comfort, food is simply fuel for my body.

Eating Trances

Record whether or not the following activities cause you to mindlessly munch. If they do, what do you tend to eat?

Watching television

At the movies

Out with friends

Shopping

At family gatherings

At social events

At business events

In the car

While reading

On coffee breaks

At sporting events

At holiday gatherings

Other

Food Triggers and Cues to Eat

When you are changing your eating patterns and habits, you want to become aware of the triggers or cues of your old patterns. A trigger is the cue that sets your pattern in motion. It could be as simple as seeing the time on the clock and thinking, "Oh, it's time for coffee." Think about 12:00 noon, what time is that? For most people it is lunchtime. Are you hungry or simply eating out of habit because you have conditioned yourself to do so? An easy way to break a habit is by avoiding the trigger.

Become aware of these triggers and break your pattern by doing something else instead. For example, replace emotional eating with a brisk walk, a bubble bath, or the "Freedom Formula" discussed in this book. Do this consciously until you have conditioned the new pattern at an unconscious level. You will feel much better overall and you will have formed a new habit.

Your Assignment:

Notice and list the triggers and cues that tell you it is time to eat.

Location: places, parents' home, etc

Activities: board games, movies, etc

People: friends, family, and co-workers

Occasions: holidays, birthdays, parties, etc

Senses: Seeing an ad, smells and tastes that stimulate your desire to eat

Time: When is your body conditioned to eat

Mood: boredom, sadness, anger, etc

Interrupting Your Pattern

Now that you are aware of emotional eating, trances and triggers like the cookies calling you. It is time to take back control over food. You will lose control if you continue down this path. You can never have enough of what you can't have, so this cycle can cause a real problem with overeating, gaining weight, then guilt and anger – which leads to overeating, gaining weight, more guilt, more anger. Sound familiar?

This pattern must stop now – today, at this very moment. Not tomorrow, not after lunch. Right now. You will need to disturb the routine that leads to over-indulging. First clean out your kitchen. Throw out the goodies and tempting foods. If this is too painful, give it away. Pack it all up and run out of your house to your closest neighbor and say, "Save me from this! You can throw it out if you don't want it." This works. Sure they think your nuts, but eventually they will wish they had your attractive physique. You must clean out all of the junk even if you have kids. Tell them they need a break from the junk as well.

Now you need a back-up plan. Sit down for five minutes and plan your eating schedule. Know on Monday what you will eat on Friday. This will help you tremendously. It is not exciting but it works. I snack on the same food every day but when I put on a pair of pants that were tight and I don't have to suck in my stomach to zip them up, it is worth it. Plan it all out. It is the only way to break a pattern of over eating. Because planning your meals and being prepared will replace your old impulsive eating trance. You are interrupting the old behavior on a regular basis until it is no longer an option. You have a new behavior instead.

You will need to go to the grocery store or the farmers' market to stock your kitchen with healthy snacks and protein drinks. Make a list and stick to the list. I suggest starting with string cheese, nuts, celery, cucumbers, baby carrots, protein drinks, eggs, apples, soy chips, spinach and some healthy low fat lean cold cuts. Tell your family and supportive friends that you have decided to make your health a priority.

My husband has heard me say at least a hundred times: "I have to get 50 more years out of this body and that means eating healthy and exercising, what I need from you is…"

Tell them how to help you. Trust me, this works too. Sure they will think you're odd but at this point, who doesn't? The last thing you need to worry about is what everyone thinks about you. All that matters is you're being true to yourself. I believe God created us to do something amazing with our lives. You need a healthy body to do that amazing "something."

Stay focused on you and your health, not whose feelings you will hurt if you don't taste their special high calorie, artery clogging, life shortening dish. Just say, "I am not hungry right now, but it looks delicious," or, "Oh my goodness, look at the time! Excuse me for a moment…"

Instead of eating out of habit or to deal with emotions, become aware of your trigger and cue to eat, and replace the old patterns with a new one. Plan ahead and be prepared. Take the time to decide a healthier more appropriate alternative. You are in control of food. You have choices.

Your Assignment:

List some of the "patterns" that need to change and an alternative.

Old Pattern	New Pattern
I snack on chips after work.	*I precut vegetables to snack on.*

The Committee

Have you thought at times "I won't lose weight," or, "If I do lose weight, I will only gain it back"? I call those limiting thoughts "the committee."

The committee is filled with well meaning members who are voicing their opinions about you and your choices. Who sits on your committee? Based on my experience it is most likely your family, friends and various people who have left an impression on you, both good and bad. I have also noticed those who have judged you harshly often reside on the committee. Most of these members were not invited to participate, they simply have "shown" up.

If you received consistent positive feedback when you were young, then as an adult you probably are confident and have high self-esteem. If this is the case you have some healthy members on your committee.

If however you received a fair amount of negative feedback as a child, you might feel self-doubt as an adult. In this case you may have some brutal members on your committee.

Beliefs are powerful. They dictate how you conduct your life. These beliefs are echoed in the feedback from your committee.

Empowering beliefs which represent your positive committee members encourage you to pursue your goals. They are the reason you stay focused because somewhere within you is the belief that you will succeed.

The negative ("realistic") members on your committee usually have negative comments that can easily discourage you. I call this negative feedback 'limiting beliefs.' Limiting beliefs try to help you, but often hold you back.

For example, when I was young my mother often commented on how attractive she was before she had children. Saying, "I remember when I was thin..." or, "You wait until you have children, you'll gain weight." My mother always struggled with her weight. So I had some committee members who were convinced I, too, would struggle, after having children. Now fast-forward to my gaining about 50 pounds when I was pregnant. I unconsciously believed this theory to be true. But at the same time I consciously wanted to return to my ideal weight.

As a result of this conflict with my belief system, there were subtle ways I found to manifest my fears, such as not making time to exercise or overindulging in sweets. When I noticed my waistline had not returned, the first thing I thought was, "See, my mother was right, once you have children, the weight just piles on." When I recognized that this was a limiting belief on my committee, I dismissed it immediately and replaced it with one that I found empowering. Once you understand this process, you will be free to choose the beliefs on your committee.

The steps to changing a belief:

1. **Identify the limiting belief.** (*my body will never be the same after having children*)

2. **Explore what its purpose is for you.** (*to feel close to and loved by my mother*)

3. **Find another way to meet that need.** (*establish an authentic, nurturing relationship with women*)

4. **What is holding you back from meeting this need?** (*fear that women will feel threatened by me if I am attractive*)

5. **Decide what you would like instead.** (*have close relationship with women WHILE feeling attractive*)

6. **Create an empowering belief that supports your need and your desired outcome.** (*I am an attractive mom who has many nurturing women friends.*) Look for examples to support your Thinking Thin Thought. When you meet a woman who is like this, add her to you committee.

7. **Condition it until it becomes automatic.** Whenever you notice the old belief surfacing you need to **STOP** and replace it with your Thinking Thin Thought: "*I am an attractive mom who has many nurturing women friends...*" Remember: never, ever, give up.

Limiting Beliefs on Your Committee

Based on what you have just learned, let's meet some of your committee members. List the members on your committee who are not supporting you. Then list their purpose for you, trust your intuition on this, it is very common that what they want for you is positive yet what they say is negative.

Your Assignment:

To elicit your limiting beliefs and list them below.

Committee members: Limiting belief member represents   Purpose

Mom   Mom's are supposed to gain weight   Love & Protection

Empowering Beliefs to Add to Your Committee

When eliminating a limiting belief it is wise to replace it with an empowering one. If you don't do this you will have a vacancy on your committee. That means it is up for grabs and usually the most dominant personalities take over. It is not a good idea to leave an empty seat on your committee. The media is working night and day to influence you, which means if a problem arises you might find yourself echoing the words from your favorite character on a TV show. Sure it is funny, but is it in your best interest?

The one that drives me crazy is when my children do something unexpected and out of the blue and I just hear my mothers words come out of my mouth. Where did that come from? I work so hard to be different, yet under stress we regress. So plan ahead, pick new positive members and invite them to be on your committee. Ask yourself how they would handle a situation, what are their thoughts about this topic. If is resonates than adopt it if not get curious on how to develop a belief that will fit your personality and empower you.

Think of a person who represents a belief or philosophy that would easily allow you to change your perspective. You can identify this by reading books about people or observing people who have traits you admire. When I was exploring my limiting beliefs about being a mother and being attractive, I wanted to find role models of this. My RAS was at work looking for me, because one day I turned on the TV and there was Goldie Hawn. I have always liked Goldie Hawn, she is funny, intelligent, attractive and an adoring mother. I watched her on TV with her daughter Kate Hudson and she beamed while Kate spoke. I thought to myself, "Boy she looks so good, she is just adorable, she seems like she gets better with time," and BINGO the light went off! I realized she needs to be on my committee. This is how your mind works, it seeks what you are looking for.

Your Assignment:

List positive people or philosophies on your committee and your Thinking Thin Thought that is a direct result on having their presence known.

New members on committee: **New empowering belief:**

Goldie Hawn   *Mom's are youthful, fun and loved by all!*

Identifying Your Needs

People who are overweight are often incredibly compassionate people. In fact, they can be so tuned into the needs of others that they deny their own needs. Sometimes this is the problem – they have forgotten they have needs.

I was raised to take care of everyone but myself: I am the oldest of four and female. In an Italian family that means, "You can't do enough." Now I am not complaining, it is comical when I look back on it. But I was judged based on my efforts and how much I did to make everyone's life comfortable. The message was, "Love everyone else, sacrifice yourself or else you are being selfish."

We all have needs and desires. They allow us to feel happy, even at peace with ourselves. When we neglect our needs we will feel empty, resentful, unfulfilled. People have difficulty identifying their needs. A healthy self-image is the result of knowing yourself well enough to meet your needs.

Assignment:
Identify your top seven needs and rank them in order of importance.

Be Accepted	Feel Accomplished	Be Acknowledged	To Feel Organized
To Feel Loved	To Be Right	To Feel Cared For	To Feel Productive
To Feel Safe	To Be in Control	To Be Creative	To Have Freedom
To Be Busy	To Be Comfortable	To See Beauty	To Communicate
To Feel Heard	To Feel Powerful	To Be Honest	To Have Order
To Belong	Be True to Myself	Recognition	To Feel Peace
To Laugh	Time Alone	To Be Different	To Be Liked
To Contribute	To Have Adventure	To Be Playful	To Nurture
To Fix Things	Make a Difference	To Feel Connected	To Have Balance
To Travel	Feel Important	To Be Affectionate	To Move (body)

Honoring Your Needs

Now that you are aware of your needs, it is important to honor them. This means to make yourself a priority and take the time to validate you. You deserve to spend time focused on you and your needs. List your top seven needs below and how you honor each need.

Set boundaries around this special time. Don't settle for less.

My need: **How I honor my need:**
Time alone   *Candlelit bubble bath at night.*

Rediscovering Yourself

It is amazing how quickly we can lose ourselves in life. I was raised to base my value on what I do for others. This is true for many of us, not just women. The more we give of ourselves the more valuable we feel. It is the main way we create our identity.

We define ourselves based on our role as a mother/father, daughter/son, sister/brother, grandmother/grandfather, wife/husband, and boss/employee. You are more than the role you play, you are so much more than that! In order to identify the true you, the question must be asked who am I when I am not being a mother/father, daughter/son, sister/brother, wife/husband, etc.? Who am I if all of those roles were taken away? What if you are supposed to be you, who is this person?

This can be a scary thought, I know it was for me. When I was going through my divorce, early during my separation from my children's father, my children would go to their father's home for an evening or a weekend. This was good for them and him, I understood. I was grateful that my children had a father that loved them so much and made time with them a priority. But I felt empty, my purpose was gone. I had for years defined myself as a wife, then Rozetta and Regis' mom, etc. It was my total identity. I had to ask myself, "Rosa who are you? What if you didn't have kids to take care of, or a husband to help climb the corporate ladder, who in the world does God want you to be?" What would make you get out of bed tomorrow morning?"

That is when I began to explore my purpose and passion in life. That is when I began to teach classes on the days my children were away. That is how I came to discover who I really am.

Ask yourself who you are, and how can you shed those expectations of what others expect from you. We teach people how to treat us and what to expect from us based on our self image and how we define our value in this world. Spend some time with yourself and see who emerges.

Your Assignment:

Take time to be present and be the person God created you to be.

Know Your Values

People looking for help in losing weight often say "motivate me." Everyone is motivated in a different way. We learn valuable information about you when you answer the question, "What motivates you?" The answer hints at what your values are, and what you will work to gain. When your values aren't being met, you lose interest.

You can make incredible changes in your life. The path to staying focused is to live in harmony with your values. As you explore your needs they will guide you to your values. Needs are a way to fulfill your values. Ask yourself, "What does this need give me?" This will lead you to your values.

Your Assignment:

Circle and rank your top seven values. If you get stuck, think of your life without that value, if you can't then it is pretty important to you.

Love	Family	Relationships	Inner Peace	Spirituality
Security	Adventure	Balance	Freedom	Connection to Others
Creative Expression	Communication	Financial Freedom	Power	Health
Honesty	Career	Success	Be True to self	Solitude
Control	Playfulness	Humor	Travel	Learning
Be Unique	Be Accepted	Social Connection	Contribution	Happiness
Making a difference	Respect	Nature	Harmony	Express Feelings
Knowledge	Be My Best	Integrity	Feel Attractive	Beauty
Have Fun	Accomplishment			

Live in Harmony with Your Values

When you live in harmony with your Values, life seems effortless. You make decisions easily. You know how to motivate yourself, by focusing on your Values. You know what you want and why. It is vital that you find a way to honor your Values. They must be part of your everyday life.

Once you are clear on your Values, you will want to filter all your decisions through them. If they support the Value then you proceed. If they do not then it is a Distraction and you say NO! No is a complete sentence, you don't need to explain, just say no.

Your Assignment:

Write down your top seven Values and review them daily.

My Value:	How I honor this value:
Inner Peace	*Anytime I spend time alone*

Setting Your Boundaries

You have identified your needs. You have clarified your values. Now how do you create a life that honors what you need and what you value most? That requires setting your boundaries. The world isn't going to magically reorientate itself around your awareness of what is most important to you.

The opposite might happen, people will object, they will tell you, "This is the way it is, deal with it." Your family and friends don't (unconsciously) want you to change, because it would mean their lives will change. When you realize that you need some quiet time for yourself and that your Value of health hasn't been honored in years, you are going to have to make a decision. Either to continue as you've been (overweight and unhappy) or make a change. If you choose to make a change and I hope you do, you will have to find time to exercise and eat healthy.

You might decide to join a yoga class, this will meet both your need for quiet time and your value of health with at the same time. Then you have to tell your family that they are going to have to make arrangements for preparing dinner, driving to practice or doing the dishes. They may not jump for joy when they hear they have more to do, they probably like having you do so much. So you set a boundary. One that says what you are comfortable with, what you expect from others and what you will not tolerate.

I have a need for quiet time on a daily basis, when I first discovered this my children were pretty young. So I had to decide how I would meet my need, one easy way was a bubble bath at night with an aromatic candle. This is something I still look forward to. In the beginning when I first began this ritual, my daughter (who was only about two), would walk into the bathroom and play with my bubbles and wander out. I knew she was safe and considering her age, I knew that was the best I was going to get unless I waited for her to fall asleep. But years later when she learned how to answer the phone, she would come in with the phone in her hand and tell me it was for me. That is where I draw the line, I refuse to talk on the phone during my quiet time. Occasionally one of my sisters will call during this time and they are the exception to the rule. My family knows that I like my quiet time and they have learned to respect that.

This comes from years of reinforcing my expectations and not settling for less.

Your Assignment:

List some boundaries you will need to establish to honor your needs and values.

My Need/Value: **Boundary Established:**

Time alone   *No phone calls after 9:00 pm*

Strive for an 80% Approval Rating

We have talked about making your health a priority, reducing distractions, identifying and honoring your needs, making your values a priority and not deciding your value on how much you do for others. It sounds like a lot, you might wonder,"How in the world do I go about doing all of this?" Hopefully you are beginning to realize how much of your behavior is motivated by what others expect from you.

My answer is simple and trust me it really works. "Go for an 80% approval rating." I personally believe chronic dieters are all or nothing people. They either do it all right all of the time or they don't bother trying. So in essence you are striving for a 100% approval rating.

Now what if I asked you to think about this differently, instead of 100% (which is impossible by the way), decide you will be happy with 80%. If that were true for you right now, who would you say no to? Where would you draw the line, especially when it comes to people pleasing?

I know since I decided that 80% approval was good enough, I don't mind when people are not happy with my decisions. I can say, "That's okay, I don't need everyone's approval all of the time." Guess what I discovered? People really do get over it. The world doesn't collapse, relationships don't end, and kids don't scream "I hate you -- you're evil!" (at least not yet). I have internally decided and say aloud, "This is me, I am the only (mom, wife, daughter) you have, sorry if I am not doing what you want, but this is all I have to give to you right now."

They deal with it and I take care of me. This is a good thing. Now if you feel guilty...you are doing this right. Good people who want 100% approval ratings feel guilty on a daily basis, for things that they have nothing to do with. So if you feel guilty for having your family prepare their own meal, or because you went to the gym instead of working 10 hours, I say feel the guilt and do it anyway. Trust me it passes.

This really comes in handy when you are raising teenagers. I recall when my teenage daughter (who is a gem), was upset about her prom. She wanted to go to the after prom party and I was questioning the plans. I told her I would make a decision after I spoke to the parents who would be hosting the party.

She wanted an answer immediately and she wanted it to be "yes", she said "I just want my prom to be perfect." Now I had never gone to a prom and I wanted it to be perfect for her. I missed out on my childhood, because of this I let my children fully enjoy theirs. So I tend to feel guilty if I think I am not making my kids happy 100% of the time. This is obviously not possible and they don't know what is in their best interest. But they do know my hot buttons and don't hesitate to push them to reach their outcome.

My breakthrough came as a mother, when I realized and said, "I will not be pressured into allowing you to do something that I think will not be in your best interest. I will speak to the parents and then make a decision. If that means you are unhappy with me right now I can live with that." It all worked out fine, she was able to attend the party and I felt as though I made a well informed decision. This has become my mantra for raising teenagers, "If this is the worst thing you can complain about concerning your childhood, I can live with that." Feel free to borrow it for your own belief system, it works wonders for me.

The Power of Your Words

Your life is a reflection of the thoughts you think on a consistent basis. Are you thinking healthy thoughts or negative self-defeating thoughts? To really make a change in your habits and manage your emotions and feelings you will want to learn how to change you inner dialogue. This is accomplished by selecting words and phrases that create optimism and certainty within you. The words you choose mean everything and dictate your outlook in every situation. This is a powerful shift that once you apply it to your life will literally transform your perception of the world.

Let's look at how to specifically integrate this concept into your life. You must verbatim say the word or phrase to yourself and see how you feel. Here is my example: I heard myself say to a friend: "When it comes to food I can be neurotic, I don't let myself deviate too far from my plan." Now she is very well read and in a similar profession as myself, she too has lost weight and kept it off for years. Her response was: "I don't think of it as neurotic, I am vigilant about my health, my weight and how I eat." I thought what a great word "vigilant" it creates a whole different perspective.

Try this, say to yourself: "I have to watch the white flour and sugar, I am neurotic that way." See how you feel, what are you hearing within your mind, like you are a fanatic perhaps? Who wants to be a fanatic?

Now say to yourself: "I avoid white flour and sugar, it is so bad for my body, and I am vigilant about taking care of my health." A whole different feeling, self-talk changes, empowers you and effortlessly manages your emotions. Start today to change those specific words and phrases to empower you. When the scale goes up 3 pounds, don't say, "I gained 3 pounds" say, "This is only temporarily." The meaning of the sentence has to change when you change the words.

The distinction here is to change the word that is negative or self-sabotaging to a word that empowers you. Instead of "this is hard," "this is challenging," or better yet, "this is interesting." Change, "I am struggling" to "I am learning." Instead of "low carb," say, "adequate carbs." Change, "it will take a long time to lose weight" to "it is only a matter of time and I will lose the weight."

Change "Cheating" to "Indulgence":

What I am saying is that words shape our feelings.

How many times have you used the term "cheating" to describe eating? To be honest with you when I began to think thin, I never called eating - cheating. It was just "eating", as I became swept up in the carb counting world I started to think differently. Once my daughter heard me refer to an indulgence as a "sinful treat" (ouch) as she said no, that is just a "guilty pleasure". I thought well that sounds better than sinful. Then I thought, what would be ideal, perhaps an indulgence? How do you refer to food? What words are you using?

This is where our vocabulary once again will influence the rest of our day. Compare a healthy indulgence to cheating. If you "cheated" then you would be feeling "bad" about food, but a healthy indulgence means you didn't do any real damage.

Listen to the words you choose, this will demonstrate if your subconscious mind's self-talk is empowering or self defeating. Naturally thin people had empowering self-talk concerning food daily. They rarely listen to it consciously, but if you asked them, "What are you thinking about this cake right now?" They would respond with something like: "Honestly, store bought cake doesn't do anything for me." How boring is that? Who wants to eat after thinking that? Try saying it to yourself, I have, and I find the cake less appealing. Now this isn't my thought, I couldn't come up with a thought like that to save my life. I borrowed it from one of my naturally thin friends.

Your Assignment:

Be mindful of your self-talk, change the words you are choosing to empower you. This is out of your awareness, you do it unconsciously. Now it is time for you to notice! Discuss it with your support team.

You Co-Create Your Reality

I am a master practitioner of NLP (neuro linguistics programming). It is the study of the mind / neurological connection. One area we really haven't discussed is being at cause. It is an NLP term we use. In order to successfully work with a client an NLP practitioner is taught to only work with a client who is at cause. That means they realize they are the cause of the problem and they are the cause of the solution. Problems are created in an unresourceful state of mind. The solution exists, in order to access it you must be in a resourceful state of mind. Therefore since we are creating the problem, we can create the solution.

This usually gets quite a rise out of people when I bring it up, but hear me out, think about it, talk about it online or with your team and see how you feel. Change can only occur when you are at cause, this is true for every person, myself included.

Ask yourself, what is my biggest challenge with creating a healthy lifestyle? What is the cause of this challenge? If the answer is outside of yourself then you cannot change it. You only have control over yourself, no one else. But I am going to ask you to change your perspective to put yourself at cause so that you can change.

Let me give you an example. I am very busy, I don't have time to exercise. Why? Because I work, run my business, take my kids to school, to their activities, some mornings I have meetings at 7:00 am and I may not return until 6:00 PM. Then I will have more running around to do, plus prepare dinner, answer emails and phone calls, etc. I am sure this sounds familiar. But if I said that's the problem… everyone else, then I have no choice, I am not accepting that I am the cause of my problem (not exercising).

How can I be at cause, the answer is easy, I don't make time for me. I say yes to everyone except myself. How can I change this? By deciding I have ability to solve this and make time for exercise, and I deserve it. I sat down with my family and said "I need time," who can help me prepare dinner or give my son a ride or pick up some groceries, etc.

I am not asking for permission, I am informing everyone of my intention. Now I have everyone pitching in, being sensitive to the fact that I have unmet needs.

Since doing this, I have formed an alliance with two of my neighbors, we work out every morning at 5:30. I have always had time at that hour and I feel better for the entire day. My family is impressed with my dedication and has been helping me even more in others areas because they know how important my workout is to me. When you take responsibility to find your solutions, it trickles into other areas of your life as well. We are holistic beings and everything is connected.

The point is that you have to realize that you are creating your life. When something isn't the way you want it to be you must ask yourself, what do you need to do to create what you want. This is true empowerment. I know this for a fact, I wouldn't be here today if I didn't put myself at cause for overcoming some terrible situations. I have survived abusive relationships, betrayal and adversity. It would have been easy for me to be a victim and blame others for my life, but what would that do other than give me more of the same.

Instead I decided to be at cause and take back control over my life and change my perspective until I found one that created my desired outcome. I know this is a heavy topic but it is vital for your long-term success. I care about you and I want to see you create a healthy long and happy life.

Your Assignment:

Ask yourself how you are at cause and how you can create what you want. Remember your life depends on it.

Thinking Thin Thought:
"I am at cause in my life, I am actively co-creating my reality."

Manage your State…of Mind

Since we are looking at ourselves and realizing that we are at cause, we will need to ask ourselves how to stay in a resourceful and proactive state of mind. It is in this mindset that the answers to our problems will surface. I always say weight management is thought management. It is the art and science of managing your mind's thoughts to motivate you to stay on track and create a healthy body. Managing your state of mind means choosing your emotions. Here are two definitions I found in dictionary.com:

Emotion:
1. A mental state that arises spontaneously rather than through conscious effort and is often accompanied by physiological changes;
2. A psychic and physical reaction (as anger or fear) subjectively experienced as feeling and physiologically involving changes that prepare the body for action

In other words you are not CHOOSING your emotions they are randomly "popping" into your head and leaving you with a SUBJECTIVE feeling. A false feeling because it isn't authentic, it is based on your biased perception.

Based on this definition, feelings result from your emotions. You are not your feelings, you simply have feelings. They come and go, within moments they can change. It all depends on your state of mind at the time and how you filter information in that moment. Just imagine that you are looking for your wallet and can't find it. How do you feel? Now imagine that the last time you saw it was last night at a restaurant and you set it down on the table. How do you feel? Now think for a moment and realize that all of your credit cards, driver's license and a spare key to your home were in your wallet. How do you feel? Now imagine you run out to your car hoping you dropped it in the car…open the door… (how do you feel?). Look under the driver's seat and there it is. How do you feel? Now imagine that you look inside and see everything is still intact, but you notice a lottery ticket (the scratch off kind) you forgot all about. Scratch it off and see that you've won $10,000! How do you feel?

Feelings change depending on what your mind is focusing on. I am encouraging you to manage your mind by managing your emotions, focusing on the fun, enjoyable ways that you can create a healthy body.

People say to me "I am bored with eating the same food," I respond: "Naturally thin people don't get bored from eating the same food." Think about it. We all eat the same foods, we don't vary our diets that much, we all have about a dozen meals we eat over and over again. If eating cereal never bothered you before 4 out of 5 days then why would an omelet be any different? It's all how you label it. Instead of thinking "I have to eat the same boring foods," say: "I choose to eat the foods I eat, I like the convenience of it." Ponder the difference when you say each sentence.

You have the power to determine how you feel by managing your emotions – it all comes back to your beliefs, choosing healthy, empowering ones to build on. Why this is so important is because you take action based on your emotions, they determine what you will do. Consistent action will result in manifestation. If you believe exercise is fun, your emotions will render feelings of excitement and anticipation. You will make time to exercise and taking this action on a daily basis will result in a fit body. Which will reinforce and further strengthen your belief, exercise is not only fun but it is fulfilling. Naturally thin people don't listen to their emotions, they unconsciously manage their state and take action until they manifest the result that is supporting their belief.

Your Assignment:

Practice managing your state of mind, remember: Beliefs lead to emotions. Emotions lead to actions. Actions taken consistently result in Manifestation.

What do you need to believe to manifest a healthy, trim body? What emotions will support this belief? What actions will you take based on this state of mind? What will you manifest once you have consistently applied this pattern?

It is All About Balance

When I see someone struggling to lose weight I will often see that they are out of balance in some area of their lives. It can be physically, emotionally and / or nutritionally. It is my belief that balance is the key to every area of our lives. When a client is not losing weight I explore areas that could be out of balance.

Some questions to ask yourself are:

1. Is there an area of my life that I need to let go of? It might be symbolic of our own weight holding, we need to let go of the weight, yet we hold on. If this is true, start with simple "letting go" tasks, such as cleaning out closets, getting rid of clutter. The subconscious mind is symbolic, it perceives events differently than the conscious mind.

2. Is there an area of my life that I need to restore balance? When you begin to take back control over your life you will take back control over food. A few recommendations I have for this is to make time to pray, meditate and exercise. It restores you quickly.

3. Am I unconsciously upset about something but don't feel safe or comfortable talking about it? In this case you will stuff those emotions with food. To address this, talk to someone and write in your journal.

4. Is my body weak, tired or just not feeling energized? This could be due to nutritional imbalance. If this is true, you can test it with a simple (but extensive) nutrient survey and pH testing. It can help you determine what you are lacking and how to correct it.

Your Assignment:

Communicate with your team about how you can create balance. This is not a time to complain about your life. Limit "complaining" time and move the discussion to what you can do to create more balance. Practice the "Freedom Formula" to help you relax.

Your Definition of Success

In this journey of life, we pursue many goals. Perhaps when you were a teenager you wanted your driver's license and a car, and with it, the freedom to come and go as you pleased. If freedom was an important value to you, then you would have been motivated to do whatever was required to get that license and car.

Later, after college and settling down, you may have wanted a home of your own, to honor your value of security and independence. You might have discovered once you were gainfully employed that you wanted to achieve a highly paid position. This would honor your value of success and status.

Our values in life change depending on our experiences and our maturity. That is why it is important to know our values and understand how achieving them helps us to feel successful in life.

I value wisdom, or that inner understanding of what is and what isn't, without the need for exterior approval. Wisdom for me leads to inner peace and feeling connected to my creator. It is my belief that inner peace is what we long for. When I feel inner peace I feel successful.

I am asking you to consider your definition of success. How do you know you are successful at what you do, in any area of your life including your weight and body? If it requires affirmation from outside of you, then you are giving someone else with your happiness, and ultimately your inner peace.

When I measured my value based on my family's approval growing up, I felt inadequate no matter what I did. Years later, I decided to redefined success based on my values and everything changed. I no longer needed their approval. When I stopped giving my power to others I was truly free. I could feel loved and fulfilled just sitting in my backyard. I am inviting you to stop giving away your power as well. I am offering you a way to liberate yourself from this crazy world and its dysfunctional definition of success. I learned a long time ago that if I measured my success based on how others felt about me, or even based on how many of my clients lost weight, I would have an opportunity to feel like a failure every day. I knew I was well trained and could help people, but in the end they alone had to take action.

I decided that as long as my methods are effective (which means they work when someone follows through with them), and I do my best at presenting them, then I am successful.

In my life I wear many hats, as do many of us. People ask me, "Rosa how do you do it all?" I respond with, "I have changed my definition of success." I am actually happy with myself when I am not perfect. I used to try so hard to get it right, be everything to everybody – cooked, cleaned, worked, you name it – I could do it all and do it well. But, boy was I exhausted! I found myself carrying this same expectation when I was trying to lose weight. I would feel like a failure daily. I realized that it was time to stop being so self-critical and stop comparing myself to someone else and only compare myself to myself.

I redefined success. In this new world if I eat chocolate, life goes on. If I skip a workout, I don't beat myself up about it. Now don't misunderstand this to mean I don't care or I've given up. I get right back on track; I just don't use getting off track as an excuse to feel badly about myself.

Your Assignment:

Explore the areas that you need to redefine:

Do you make yourself feel guilty if you have a treat?

Do you become moody because the number on the scale went up?

Do you feel anxious if you try hard and still don't lose weight?

Look at your answers to these questions; if you have more opportunities to feel inadequate than successful you have some decisions to make.

Pick a plan that is empowering you, your values and your outcome. This is a wonderful way to uncover empowering Thinking Thin Thoughts that will help you to redefine success. You will be on this journey for awhile. You may as well make it a pleasant one. With this mindset you won't be frantically trying to lose weight, you will be designing a life!

Instead: ask yourself questions like:

How can I have fun in this process?

What do I have to believe is true for me to feel successful on a daily basis?

How can I stop comparing myself to others and only to myself?

Who can support me best on this journey?

The Body:

Your Diet Personality

I have been a student and a teacher of the Enneagram, which studies nine styles of expression. People like people who they relate to and learning about personality styles allows us to understand those types that are different than ourselves. I like teaching personality styles to couples because it can really deepen a relationship when two people realize that their mate is only being who they are suppose to be. The person God intended them to be, they aren't trying to be difficult, they just perceive the world differently than we do and have formed a way of "being" to adjust to their perceived reality.

What I found was that when you are pointing out someone's flaws in their personality styles you have to be a bit careful not to hurt their feelings. What I decided to do is have fun with these styles, since we all have flaws and gifts. We learn quite a bit from being honest about our "dark side". To accomplish this I created a series of characters and poked fun at the styles by exaggerating their flaws. Participants would laugh and then admit that yes, it was true, they were "Tyrone the Taskmaster" and ask for suggestions for improvement. In the same vain, I decided to create diet personality styles that would help you do the same thing. They are based on the common reasons people are overweight. They are not gender specific, go through the checklist and then read the explanation that follows. I have an online version located on MindOverPlatter.com (http://www.mindoverplatter.com/freeDietPersonalityQuiz.php).

The styles are Fast-Paced Freddy, Low-Fat Laura, Over-Eating Oscar and Carb-Addict Carla. Check all the boxes that apply to you on a consistent basis then tally up the totals. You will more than likely be a blend of styles, this is common. It will give you direction on where you will want to focus first to manage your weight.

Your Assignment:

Take the Diet Personality Quiz: There is no right or wrong answer.

Fast Paced Freddy:

- □ I often skip meals.
- □ I eat a large dinner and often snack into the evening.
- □ I am usually in a hurry.
- □ I eat in my car at times or while on the move.
- □ I rarely plan my meals
- □ I eat fast food on a regular basis.
- □ If I eat breakfast, it is something quick.
- □ I can go all day without eating.
- □ I eat the bulk of my food intake after 3:00pm.
- □ I become very hungry in the evening / night.

_____ Total

Over Eating Oscar:

- □ I dine at places that serve large portions.
- □ I have a habit of cleaning my plate.
- □ I have a big appetite.
- □ I don't like to be restricted.
- □ I think about food all day.
- □ I find it hard to stop eating once I start.
- □ I won't follow a strict diet.
- □ I feel guilty wasting food.
- □ I feel sluggish mid afternoon and take a coffee & cookie break.
- □ I love meat, potatoes and pasta.

_____ Total

Carb Addict Carla:

- I am hungry shortly after eating breakfast.
- I have intense cravings for sweets/bread/pasta, etc
- I have a difficult time losing weight.
- I have not lost weight following a low fat diet.
- I often feel tired after lunch / late meals.
- I crave sweets especially after a meal.
- I tend to retain water.
- Once I start to eat sweets, I crave more.
- I feel sluggish mid afternoon and take a coffee & cookie break.
- I have mood swings if I don't eat when I am hungry.

_____ Total

Low Fat Laura:

- I usually have a healthy breakfast.
- I typically have soup and salad for a meal.
- I try to exercise on a regular basis.
- I snack on low fat foods.
- I strive for 5 fruits and vegetables daily.
- I eat pasta, rice or grains for dinner.
- I cook low fat and healthy for most of my meals.
- I have been eating low fat for years.
- When I eat sweets I eat a low fat version.
- I feel hungry throughout the day.

_____ Total

Fast Pace Freddy:

About you:

If you rated high in this area then you are probably a mover and a shaker. You are a very busy person with a fast paced lifestyle. This could be great for your career but damaging to your body. Most Freddy's are not only over weight but are prone to high blood pressure, heart disease and anxiety. This in part is due to the high fat, sodium, sugar and calorie foods that are convenient yet harmful with daily consumption. This coupled with the type A personality style will accelerate health problems and weight gain.

What is happening:

What is happening is that you are consuming foods that are not good fuel sources. This means your body is STARVING for nutrition. You might be overweight but chances are good you are undernourished. The other problem with the fast pace of Freddy is that you don't have time to eat, so you skip meals and wait until you are famished to eat. Once you do eat, you lose control and consume too much. This many calories at one time are too much for the body to process. The majority will be stored for fuel, to be burned within a few hours. But if you go to sleep or relax your body will convert the excess fuel into fat.

Another dynamic that is occurring due to being so busy is the over stimulation of your adrenal glands which will provoke cortisol being released. This is a natural response when we need to fight or flight, but not healthy when continuously activated. In other words, consistent stress exhausts adrenal glands and causes us to run on adrenalin, which in turn tells the body we are in "survival mode". This alerts cortisol to be produced telling our body to prepare for a famine. The body protects you by increasing your fat reserves around the belly, hips and thighs. This is hard wired into our system, the body wants to live, and has mechanisms in place to ensure it for as long as possible.

What to do:

First begin to plan ahead. If you are going to be busy then you must accept the fact that life is busy and you are going to need to eat. Plan your meals in advance. Decide what you are going to eat for breakfast, lunch and dinner. Go to the store and purchase a small insulated cooler bag, some plastic zip lock sandwich bags, bottles of water, veggies, string cheese, almonds, soy chips, protein bars and drinks. Then pack snack size portions for your car and nibble throughout the day. Then you won't be famished at dinner time.

You will also need to know where you can stop for fast food and where you should avoid. Donut shops avoid, unless they serve salads. If you are going to stop in a fast food restaurant be sure they have salads and grilled chicken. Plan 20 minutes to sit down and eat, take some deep breaths and enjoy your meal.

As far as the stress in your life, it is vital you give your adrenal glands a break. Cut back on caffeine, give yourself time to get things done, and take some good supplements. I will cover this in the chapter entitled "Supplements and Weight Loss."

If you have been eating this way for a long time I would recommend you detoxify your body. Toxins are stored in the fatty deposits and will sabotage weight loss. Once you eliminate the toxins your fat cells will be more receptive to shrinking and you will lose weight. This topic is discussed in the chapter: "Detoxify you Body".

The bottom line:

Slow down, plan ahead and follow the nine habits of naturally thin people. Pay particular attention to habit three and four. Take your time, enjoy your food and listen to your body. Chances are good you are ignoring your body's signals because you are too busy. Eat when you are hungry and stop when you are satisfied. This may mean you will need to eat a few more times a day. Even if it is a healthy snack size portion, it will fire up your metabolism and you will lose weight.

Over Eating Oscar:

About you:

If you identified with Oscar, then you know you enjoy food. You are one of those people who once you begin to eat, you can't stop. You eat healthy foods, just too much of it. You are always trying to manage your appetite and it often gets the best of you. Most Oscars love to cook, and appreciate "good" food.

Food is in control of your life. Even your entertainment is centered around food. You like buffets, want to get your money's worth and are a card carrying member of the "clean your plate" club. When you do successfully lose weight, it is often due to exercise. If you were athletic growing up your appetite hasn't been a problem because you needed the food for fuel and you naturally managed your weight. Now that your life is busier but not physically active the weight is getting harder to manage.

You probably notice an inconsistency of energy throughout the day due to fact that your body is running on either empty or full. This can really vary from day to day depending on how many meals you have skipped then overcompensated for.

What is happening:

You are not listening to your body. You are ignoring its signals for hunger until you become famished. Then you are so hungry that you overeat. Your body can not possibly burn the calories at the same ratio as you are consuming them. Your stomach is only the size of your clench fist. You don't need a large amount of food for fueling your body. This results in the majority of your food intake being stored for fat instead of being used for fuel. You are basically overloading your system with more calories and/or carbohydrates than it needs to fuel your body.

Your heart could be overstressed from the extra weight. Your liver and digestion system are overworking to process the concentration of so many calories in such a short time period, especially if you are eating your largest meal at night. The body needs to repair at night not digest food.

The diet experts tell you to eat breakfast to lose weight, yet when you do it makes you hungrier. Then you tend to eat more throughout the day as a result. Your suspicion is correct that once you start eating you feel hungrier throughout the day. This is in part due to what you are eating, it is more than likely triggering your blood sugar and causing you to feel hungry shortly there after.

What to do:

Don't force yourself to eat, but do get in the habit of a protein drink to stabilize your blood sugar first thing in the morning. You will need to properly balance your macronutrients each time you eat to satisfy your hunger and not overeat. This is discussed in the chapter entitled: "Avoid an Insulin Response".

In order for you to lose weight, you will need to eat smaller meals spaced out during the day. By properly balancing your food intake you will feel satisfied with less food. You would benefit greatly from using a Food Journal. Record what you eat as well as how hungry you are. Habit number three is essential for you, "Eat only when you are hungry and stop when you are satisfied." This is going to take you time to integrate, but hang in there, it will be the way you lose weight while enjoying some of your favorite foods.

The bottom line:

Stop having a love affair with food. It is only fuel for your body, nothing more, nothing less. Listen to your body, it knows when you are hungry and when you are full. Cut every portion in half and notice how you feel 20 minutes after you eat. Remember food is available 24 hours per day.
Overeating is only a habit, there doesn't need to be a deep-seated psychological reason for it. Just start a habit of eating small portions.

Carb Addict Carla:

About you:

Carla, Carla, Carla, I feel your pain, you crave foods like sweets, chips, pasta, bread and potatoes. You love foods that are high in starchy carbohydrate. You like how they make you feel satisfied. Sometimes too full, you may even begin to notice how bloated you are after eating certain meals that are high in carbs.

If you do give in to this "indulgence" you feel famished within an hour or two. When you have a "big" meal that is high in carbs like a pasta dinner you feel so tired that you could take a nap. As much as you know these foods are not your best choice, you love them. It is hard for you to resist the temptation of cookies, sweets, breads, potatoes, etc. Even if you just ate, you always have room for dessert. It's like an addiction.

Your best successes in weight loss have been when you cut down drastically on starchy carbohydrates. When you think about it, you felt great and didn't even miss the pasta. You had energy and you were in a good mood consistently. But for some reason, once the weight came off you thought you could return to your old eating habits.

It started innocently with a piece of pie or cake then you wanted ice cream, the next day you craved mashed potatoes and it went down hill from there. When you woke up in the morning with a carb hangover you thought, "I must be coming down with something." So you had a bagel to settle your stomach, then it was pizza day at the office and you forgot lunch. If you relate to this then it is time to change. The first step to change is with awareness, your body reacts to carbs, plain and simple.

What is happening:

You are having a physical reaction to sugar. I wrote "Avoid an Insulin Response" for you. Your blood sugar is on a roller coaster ride. As a result you are more than likely provoking an insulin response many times during the day. This can cause your body to produce fat even if you are not eating a lot of calories.

What to do:

You have to change your lifestyle to incorporate the fact that too many carbs will trigger an insulin response and you could easily lose control over your cravings.

In order for you to burn fat and lose weight you will need to manage your insulin levels. You can successfully accomplish this by properly balancing your macronutrients. But first you will want to control those sugar cravings. The best way to do that is to rebalance your body by fasting from sugar. You can accomplish this by following the eating plan outlined in "Avoid an Insulin Response."

If you are a person who likes a well outlined eating plan and wants to accelerate the process then you might want to read "The 21 Day-Diet™". It will literally train your body to use stored fat for fuel rather than sugar. You will lose weight, but I will warn you it is drastic and restricting. That is why it is for 21 days, because I want you to retrain your body to not crave sugar. I have seen people lose up to 15 pounds in 21 days following the plan.

The bottom line:

Start off each day with a protein based breakfast to stabilize your blood sugar. Have snacks available with protein like: peanuts, boiled eggs, string cheese, chicken breast, hummus, tofu, soy nuts and chips, etc. Stay away from the trigger foods that you know will cause you to lose control. Especially white flour and sugar based foods, try fasting from these foods for a week and see how you feel. Avoid eating trigger foods within the first 21 days of this program. Memorize "Naturally Thin Habit #9", the 80/20 rule; as long as you are making good choices 8 out of 10 times you are a success.

Low Fat Laura:

About you:

You tend to eat healthy meals and snack on low fat foods. You seldom "cheat" because you plan your meals ahead of time. You make time to exercise on a regular basis. You are disciplined with what you eat and how much. You know all of the dieting "tricks" like replacing butter with margarine, whole milk with skim and don't mind.

You prefer to prepare foods yourself but if you dine out, you know which restaurants will offer what fits into your eating plan. You order your dressing on the side, ask for water and move the bread basket to the other side of the table. You rarely eat rich foods or desserts and if you do only have a small portion. Overall you have healthy habits.

Your diet is balanced, eating three meals per day with a focus on watching those fat grams. You know the low fat version of almost any food. You are driven by a desire to be healthy and according to your doctor are in good health. Your friends are impressed with your vigilant focus on health. With all this effort, you don't understand why you have those extra pounds that just won't go away.

What is happening:

Your body's hormones and essential fatty acids are more than likely out of balance. When this happens the metabolism isn't functioning at its optimal rate.

With all your good intentions and the popularity of the low fat craze you have taken something good to an extreme. Your meals are not in proper balance. Now you have to restore balance by increasing the right fat. This isn't your fault, we have been "brainwashed" to believe fat is bad. But good fats are healthy for your body and will actually help you to burn fat, especially essential fatty acids. Plus they will satisfy your hunger and you will consume less food.

What to do:

Start to add fat to your diet. This will be hard for you because you are so adversely conditioned when it comes to eating fat. I recommend you begin to research the topic more, since you like to learn about health and nutrition, this will be easy for you.

You need to rebalance your body's chemistry. Begin to use extra virgin olive oil in your meals. Mix it with balsamic vinegar for salad dressing, use it in place of butter or margarine, stir-fry your vegetables in it. Have a couple of eggs in your diet, the lecithin in the yokes is actually good for you.

Try adding a couple slices of avocado and olives to your meals. I know this is going to sound crazy but snack on a handful of raw almonds. Nuts are naturally balanced by nature, they make great snacks. Nuts have protein, fat and carbs all properly balanced to not provoke your blood sugar.

In a matter of weeks you will notice a big difference in your body, not only will your lose weight, but your skin will glow and you will look more youthful. You will be amazed to discover how many foods you can eat and still lose weight.

You will definitely benefit from supplements that are outlined to restore essential fatty acids. These are outline in the chapter "Supplements and Weight Loss".

The bottom line:

Plain and simply, your body needs more fat, at least the right kind of fat. Focus on balance and essential fatty acids like ones found in omega 3, 6 and 9, try taking a tablespoon of flax seed oil daily. Foods with healthy fats include: extra virgin olive oil, peanuts, raw almonds, (all nuts and seeds), flax seeds, fish, especially salmon, eggs, peanut butter, avocados, olives etc. Follow the eating plan outlined in this book.

9 Habits of Naturally Thin People

What is a naturally thin person? In my opinion after years of observation, I consider a naturally thin person someone that would gain weight if they overate, but they don't overeat. They have successfully managed their weight for years. I have studied naturally thin people as well as chronic dieters. With my roots in hypnosis and NLP, I have become a student of the mind and its influence on the body. As unique and special as we are individually and spiritually, we follow patterns – as humans – that are very predictable. What I found in my studies is that when chronic dieters start thinking like naturally thin people they lose weight! This is how I kept off 30 pounds for years – by changing the way I think.

Naturally thin people have similar habits. Being thin comes so "naturally" to them that they are not even aware of what they are doing. When you think like a naturally thin person, you will develop the same habits. When you develop the same habits, you will reap the same results. You will be amazed at how much progress you can make as long as you stay focused and integrate these habits as part of your daily life.

When I read the latest diet book that is based on a culture of eating, I always notice many of the naturally thin habits are present. No one can claim these habits as exclusive to their diet. I can't honestly say I invented this program out of thin air. I have observed people who have what I want, they have successfully achieved an outcome on a physical level that I want to duplicate. What I did was compile the information and blend it with my expertise in the mind/body connection to integrate it in my life.

This is a common sense approach that validates our natural instincts. Watch a child eat, they live the naturally thin habits, it is life that reprograms them to clean their plates and use food to cope with stress. I invite you to take a look at children or a naturally thin person and notice how many of these habits they unconsciously follow. They aren't doing it to lose weight, it is just the way they are. This is the whole point, it must become a way of life for you, not a diet.

The 9 Habits of Naturally Thin People:

1. Empowering Self-Image:

They see themselves living in an attractive body.

2. Powerful Self-Talk:

They speak to themselves in ways that empower them.

3. Stop Dieting:

They don't diet, they simply eat food that they enjoy.

4. Don't Over Eat:

They eat only when they are physically hungry and stop when the hunger goes away.

5. Proper Food Combining:

They eat foods in the proper portions to manage their weight.

6. Food is a Source of Fuel:

They eat in proportion to how much fuel they need for their bodies.

7. Drink Water:

They are adequately hydrated and tend to drink water.

8. Active Lifestyle:

They move their bodies more than the average person.

9. 80:20 Rule:

They are on track more than off, they don't obsess about food.

Habit #1: Empowering Self-Image

Your self-image is a factor that will determine if you remain focused or find yourself struggling to stay at your ideal weight. Have you lost weight only to regain it? Are you tempted to revert to previous habits or patterns once you have reached your ideal weight? If this is true for you then you might want to take a look at your self-image, which is actually a reflection of your self-esteem and beliefs about yourself. This image reveals a lot about your life and who you "think" you are. It holds the key to how you see yourself in all aspects of your life.

Self-image is how you "unconsciously" see yourself. So it can be different than how you consciously see yourself. If your subconscious image is negative, such as "I am fat, lazy, and unattractive" then no matter what you do, you will continue to see yourself this way. The subconscious mind is your servant; therefore, it will manifest whatever you believe to be true. I tell my clients, "What you believe is true for you, is true for you."

So what is true for you? What images, ideals, or self-judgments do you secretly believe? You may wonder where this image comes from. It can come from your family members, friends, and even the media. It likely traces back to your childhood, when you were highly impressionable. Children don't filter incoming information, they are open and accepting, as they should be. Based on your perception of your own incoming messages as a child, you saw these messages as actual experiences. Based on these "experiences", your self-image was formed. This is the image that you are currently manifesting.

I believe when you change this image first, then the body will dutifully follow. This is how to make a long-lasting change that will seem like a natural process. This is why self-hypnosis can be so effective, because it can redesign your internal programming, which then changes your self-image. When this occurs, you are on the path to creating a wonderful new image. With patience, persistence, and time this new image will become a reality. Changing this image means changing your perception of a given experience and the beliefs that were formed as a result. When you change your perception you actually change your perspective, which in turn allows you to be more resourceful. You then see the situation differently, and you are in control. You feel empowered.

An effective way to change your self-image is to visualize your ideal image daily. Every morning as you wake up, imagine yourself in this healthy body. Let yourself become excited about it. Again, as you fall asleep at night, imagine this healthy body.

Your Assignment:

o   Take a few minutes to think about what your current self-image has been. Trust what comes to you.

o   Now think about what you want instead. You can create any image you'd like, so make it a good one.

o   Journal about it and discuss it with your team.

o   Take time to "visualize" this image daily.

o   Listen to a visualization CD with your Team and relax!

Thinking Thin Thought:

"A healthy fit body is my birthright!"

Habit #2: Powerful Self Talk: Power Phrase

Okay, Boss! Your thought is my command. Your self-talk is key to your success. Your brain has the ability to scan the environment to bring to your attention what you are thinking about. Therefore it is absolutely necessary that you speak to yourself in a manner that is consistent with your ultimate goals and desires.

This means saying healthy things to yourself like, "I have a healthy relationship with food," or "I am in control of food," or – and this is one of my favorites – "Food is here all day, everyday; I don't have to eat it all right now!"

Your brain is listening to every word you say to yourself 24-7. Your subconscious mind takes what you say as a direct command and responds with, "Okay, boss!" Then it alerts you when it finds what you told it to look for. If you say, "I am bored eating this way," it responds with, "Okay, boss!" Then it reminds you to focus on being bored with your food choices. If you say, "I can eat the same thing everyday and never feel bored," your subconscious mind says, "Okay, boss!" – and directs your mind to that which keeps you from feeling bored. It really works, try it for yourself. Focus on a positive statement and repeat it daily.

Sammy' Self-Image:

Sammy wanted to get into body-building. We talked about his self-image and how it compared to that of successful body-builders. He started to repeat to himself, "I am in top shape, my body is strong and fit." During this time he was at a local bookstore and he saw a book that caught his eye. A step-by-step book for beginner body builders on how to create a "chiseled" physique. The book had always been there, but now, with his new frame of mind, he saw it for the first time. That is exactly how the subconscious mind speaks to you. It listens to what you tell it and seeks out what you are looking for. Then it alerts you in many ways, through intuition, self-talk, someone else's suggestions, events that you see as 'coincidences,' and through many other channels. This is also known as the RAS that we spoke about earlier in the book. Your subconscious mind is communicating with you. The question is: are you listening?

Power Phrase Examples:

A power phrase is something you say to yourself daily, to support your goal and outcome. It is much like an affirmation or a mantra. You will want to eventually change your power phrase to an actual belief. Ask yourself, "If I really believed this, how would I act?" My clients who have used these phases have created profound life changes. Listed are some examples, which you can customize to suit you. Or you can design one specifically for you.

Your Assignment:

Repeat each statement to yourself, imagine how good it would feel to really believe that they are true for you now…

"Nothing tastes as good as a fit body feels"   "I feel healthier today than yesterday"

"My body is beautiful"   "I am fit and attractive, I look great"

"My stomach is flat and firm, I feel good"   "I always leave food on my plate"

"I eat only when I am hungry"   "I stop eating when I am satisfied"

"I am strong, healthy, and lean"   "I am perfect exactly as I am"

"I love and accept myself as I am"   "I eat healthy, small portions of food"

"I lose weight easily and effortlessly"   "My body burns food for fuel"

"My health is my number one priority"   "I am in control of food"

"Food is a source of fuel for my body"   "Food is not a source of comfort"

"I enjoy the company far more than the food"   "The less food I eat the better I feel"

Habit #3: STOP Dieting!

Aren't you sick of dieting? I know I am.

As a chronic dieter I was constantly on a diet from an early age. My mother is a great cook and when I was growing up she liked to cook traditional Italian meals from scratch. My brother, sisters, and I were expected to clean our plates every day at every meal. You didn't want to leave food on your plate around my family. It was an insult to leave food on your plate; it was a bigger insult if you didn't ask for seconds. I became an overeater from day one. I didn't mind most of the time because everything my mother made for us was delicious. Because we were poor, it was either feast or famine, this installed a fear of deprivation with me. Like most people I became a chronic dieter early in life.

I remember as a teenager when I was in my body cast, I decided to go on my first diet. I read many diet books (my mother had plenty of them). I developed a low-calorie diet and even found ways to exercise. I would go hungry for hours and was always counting calories in my head. I was determined to not gain a pound and maybe even lose a few. It worked. When my cast came off I think I weighed less than when I started. My waist was 23 inches (plaster has its advantages!). I was hooked. This was the beginning of my becoming a chronic dieter. I would either eat too much or very little. As you may have noticed by now, I had a lot of issues to overcome when it came to food and meal-time.

I didn't realize at that early age that the answer to losing weight was not found in depriving my body of food. Deprivation and starvation will create an obsession with food. This all-or-nothing thinking will magnify your obsession with food. Since you can never get enough of what you can't have, it is only a matter of time and you will over-indulge. This "forbidden" act sets you up for failure. We have all done this.

People who chronically diet think of this "forbidden" indulgence as their last meal. I call it The "Last Supper" mindset. They justify that they will get back on track tomorrow. Since they have "blown it", they may as well make it worthwhile. You know how it goes; you had a cookie, so now you may as well have the mocha latte.

Since you did that you figure, "Let's order pizza," then you think, "Well I already blew it, so I'll have a banana split and start fresh tomorrow." It's crazy, isn't it? But this is how chronic dieters think; it's all or nothing. This way of thinking leads to overeating and bingeing, not just for that one day, but as a way of life. We diet, then overeat; it's a vicious cycle. Naturally thin means moderation, eat food when you are hungry and focus on it being a source of fuel to energize your body.

Chronic dieting harms your body. It slows down your metabolism, lowers your body's muscle mass, and increases your body fat. This means you will gain weight even faster than before you began the diet. It can take as long as a year to readjust the metabolism to its pre-diet rate. This is an endless cycle that leaves you feeling hopeless, deprived, and – more likely than not, overweight. You want to strive for proper balance over the long term, a lifestyle that will burn fat and build muscle. You want to lose fat, not necessarily weight. Don't worry about the number on the scale; focus on your body fat.

Abby's Focus:

When Abby came to see me she weighed 200 pounds and was 49% body fat. She wanted to lose 75 pounds. I encouraged her to focus on her body fat number rather than the number on the scale. I told her the goal is not to diet, but to create a healthy body. I asked her to make her focus on getting her body fat under 30% as a result she would lose weight.

It took some time – over a year and a half, but she did it, and she looks great. I never said this was going to be fast, but it will be permanent. You will hear me say it over and over again, "Weight loss is a lifestyle, not an event."

Isn't it time you created a healthier body and mind? Say "goodbye" to going on diets. Begin today to eat for a healthy body. And respect your body. Learn a whole new way of eating to be thin. Adopt a new mindset that will guide you through this process. By following the steps outlined in this program you will condition your mind and body. The problem isn't weight. The problem is overeating. Overeating is when you eat when you are not physically hungry.

Your Assignment:

- Stop thinking about being on a diet.

- Start thinking about how to create a healthier body and lifestyle.

- Discuss this with your Team.

Thinking Thin Thought:

"Food is available 24 hours per day seven days per week. I choose to feed my body when I am physically hungry. I stop the moment I am satisfied."

Habit #4: Don't Over Eat

Rate Hunger 1-10

Eat only when you are physically hungry

I know I have said that not overeating and your percent of body fat are more important than actual weight. I'm using weight – for this discussion, because it is an easily understood common denominator. When the scale goes up, more than likely you are not following the habits of naturally thin people. One habit that I think has a major impact on your health and weight is eating when you are hungry and stopping the moment you are satisfied. Start by rating hunger on a scale from 1-10, (empty vs. full): one is famished, ten is stuffed.

Your body needs fuel and your stomach is like the fuel tank, it can be depleted or filled with fuel. Naturally thin people don't overeat, they don't like the feeling of being full or bloated. They only eat when they are hungry (which is a 2 on the scale) and they stop when they are satisfied (5 on the scale).

Practice listening to your body and eating only when you are physically hungry, then stop the moment you are satisfied. It is about half of what you would normally eat. One of my beliefs in restaurants is that I always get 2 meals for the price of one. They serve far too much food.

Don't let yourself feel too hungry either, it will cause you to lose control and overeat. This alone works, eating only when you are hungry and stopping the moment you are satisfied.

Your Assignment:

➢ Rate hunger from 1-10, eat only when you are at a 2 and stop when you reach a 5 or 6.

➢ Log this in your food journal.

➢ Discuss this with your team.

Habit #5: Properly Combine Food for Your Body.

Low-carb, high protein, low-fat, low-calorie which way is the best way? There isn't one answer for everyone. A diet plan will generally work ideally for 25% of the population at any given time. You will have to discover the best plan for your body type.

Your body communicates with you. Are you rushing through life, not listening to your body? Slow down, this isn't a race, take time to experiment with balancing protein, carbs, fat, and even calories. Notice how you feel, how stable is your weight? If you are experiencing a consistent weight loss and you have energy, then the balance is right for you. This is why I strongly recommend using a food journal. When you find that you are building muscle, reducing body fat, losing weight and feeling good, you want to be able to go to your journal and track what you've been eating. Your journal will be critical in mapping your recipe for success. If you haven't done so, begin to use your food journal and note your weight and how you feel.

White Flour and White Sugar

I would encourage you over the next few days to observe how your body responds to reducing or even eliminating white flour and sugar from your daily intake. White flour and white sugar are addictive drugs that will cause your blood sugar to skyrocket, fueling you with energy. Within hours your blood sugar will come crashing down leaving you hungry, tired, and craving more of the substance that started this rollercoaster effect. This recreates the sugar / starch craving and causes "killer" cravings and an intense hunger. The result is that you want to eat more of the very thing your body is reacting to. I am serious when I say it is an addiction. Not for everyone but for me as well as many of my clients. A Harvard study just announced that women on high-carb diets have a higher rate of breast cancer. It isn't all carbs that harm the body, it is the white flour and white sugar carbs (impact carbs) that you need to be aware of.

Get to know your body and its limits, then respect them. Keep your food journal to assist you. Don't spend too much time in denial, it will only lead you to gaining weight and a lot of frustration.

Face reality, talk to your friends and find a belief system that supports what is in your best interest. I am in this with you. We will be healthier in the long run.

I am a Carb Addict Carla, so I find for my body type, the 2:1 ratio (2 grams of Protein to 1 gram of Impact Carb), to be a good balance for me. It has worked for most of my Carb Addict clients as well. I will explain this further when I discuss "Avoid an Insulin Response."

Example: If a slice of rye bread is 14 grams of carbohydrate. Then have 28 grams of protein such as 4-5 ounces of chicken. I've seen this work for my clients. I don't recommend counting carbs from vegetables, only Impact Carbs (bread, pasta, rice, potatoes, sweets, corn, and peas) and high fructose carbs (fruit and juices).

Once I discovered that my body responds well to the 2:1 ratio, I naturally keep my weight within its ideal range without dieting. Naturally thin people have found a way to eat that works for them. Be sure to find a balance that works for you and make it a way of life. Since people like direction in this area, here are some of my observations with finding a good protein to impact carb ratio in relationship to your Diet Personality:

(This the break down per meal or snack)

- 2:1 (20 grams of protein to 10 grams of impact carbs) Carb Addict Carla, Over Eating Oscar, people with a slow metabolism.

- 1:1.5 (20 grams of protein to 30 grams of impact carbs) Low Fat Laura, people with a fast metabolism and / or exercise a lot.

- 1:1 (20 grams of protein, 20 grams of impact carbs) Fast Pace Freddy, Over Eating Oscar, people with an average metabolism.

Habit #6: Food is a Source of Fuel.

Your body will only burn so many calories per hour so when you reduce your portions to manageable chunks of calories, your body will burn those calories for fuel. Naturally thin people unconsciously think of food as an energy source. They find it an inconvenience to stop what they are doing to refuel their bodies. They eat to get it over with and then get back to what they were doing.

Food is simply a source of fuel, nothing more, nothing less. I teach my clients to balance their meals to properly fuel their bodies. This means a small meal of macronutrients (proteins, fats, carbs). Portion control is very important. You will gain weight if you overeat.

When I start working with a client I like to get some baseline information. Their weight is the least of my concerns. I want to know their Resting Metabolic Rate, which will tell me how many calories they burn at rest. I calculate their body fat percentage and determine how many pounds of their body are fat. I believe it is so important that I offer the service online to my members. I also recommend they go to the doctor for a blood test to determine: cholesterol, HDL, LDL, and triglycerides. We track of this information on an annual basis. I strongly encourage you to do the same. This will help you to know your body and see how it reacts to the foods you are eating.

This is why I want to know the above information. If your Resting Metabolic Rate is 1,800 then you are burning around 100 calories per hour depending on their activity level. That isn't much, if they eat a meal that is 500 calories, unless you exercise, you are not burning all of those calories. So the overage will be stored for later fuel. A simple solution is to eat small meals. Portion control works. Naturally thin people just don't overeat, they burn their incoming calories as fuel.

This is a time-tested way to managing your weight. When you munch on small meals that are properly combined, you will lose weight and your body will burn fat. You can attend picnics, parties, restaurants, family gatherings, even on vacation and sample small portions of food (properly combined) and still lose weight.

This is the habit you want to integrate in your life. This is only a habit; habits are just conditioned responses – not rocket science.

Learning something new, such as adapting a new habit, requires spatial repetition. Start today by consistently conditioning this new behavior, eating small portions of food per meal, especially when you don't feel like it. Repetition works, you need to repeat an action over and over again until it becomes an unconscious habit. You need to do this every time you eat, every meal should be a small portion and properly balanced.

What does this meal look like? As far as macronutrients and portions are concerned, you want a portion of protein (4-6 ounces is a serving), healthy fat (1 ounce is a serving), vegetables (1-2 cups), and complex carbohydrates (1/2 serving, such as 1 slice of bread, ½ fruit, ½ cup of rice or pasta).

Imagine your stomach is only the size of a clenched fist, so you don't need a lot of food for fuel. If you are not losing weight then you might be eating too much food or too much sugar based (impact carbs), calories per meal.

Your Assignment:

☐ Reduce the size of your meals to smaller servings.

☐ Write about how this feels in your journal.

☐ Discuss it with your team.

Habit #7: Drink Water

Why drink water? The topic of water and to make drinking it a priority is too important of a topic to overlook. Is this really a naturally thin habit? To be honest, I don't have the hard facts to support that a naturally thin person drinks more water than an overweight person. I have observed that naturally thin people seem content drinking water and don't resent it. They seem to choose water as a way to quench their thirst. Maybe it is because they unconsciously realized it is effectively helping them to stay hydrated. Being dehydrated is a big problem.

Considering our bodies are 55-70% water, it is a cornerstone for health. The healthier you are and the less fat you carry on your body the higher the percentage of water you have. Women tend to have a lower percent of water due to the fact that fat itself has less water than muscle. In order to maintain a level of health it is essential that you stay properly hydrated and drink plenty of water.

Water and hydration, helps regulate the body temperature, it flushes out toxins and waste from the body. There is evidence that suggests drinking adequate amounts of water will actually suppress your appetite. This is due to the fact that the body often confuses hunger with thirst. The brain receives these sensations simultaneously so we often confuse the two. Drinking a glass of water prior to eating will satisfy your thirst and reduce the desire to overeat.

Drinking 8 glasses of water a day is recommended, another theory is to take your body weight divide it in half and drink that many ounces per day of water. For example if you weigh 180 pounds then drink 90 ounces of water.

There are many studies to support that a well hydrated body experiences less pain and headaches. The brain consists of as much as 85% water. Adequate water will cushion your joints and organs, so if you suffer from back pain or arthritis, try water, it is a natural anti-inflammatory.

Many of our health problems are rooted in inflammation are the source of pain and premature aging. Avoiding an insulin response is a natural way to reduce inflammation.

Not to mention the skin is the largest organ of your body and water keeps it hydrated and smooth, youthful looking. Just compare the skin of smoker (dehydrated) to a non-smoker (hydrated) notice the difference in depth of lines and wrinkles. If you want to look 10 years younger, quit smoking and drink your water, and start to eat foods that are properly combined to avoid an insulin response.

On a completely different level, water is a carrier for not only toxins and nutrients but energy as well. Both healing energy and disruptive energy. Dr. Masaru Emoto highlights this in his book: "The Hidden Messages of Water" which was featured in the movie: "What the Bleep Do We Know." How negative and positive thoughts actually impact the molecules of water. It is a fascinating study that is well documented.

What I realized after seeing the movie and reading the study was how powerful our thoughts are coupled with the fact that our bodies are made up primarily of water, how our positive or negative thoughts affect our bodies. This point is well made in the movie which I recommend for viewing since it illustrates how the mind /body connection works in a very interesting way.

Your Assignment:
Drink eight 8 ounce glasses of water per day.

Thinking Thin Thought:

"I drink this water as a sign of my love and appreciation for myself."

Habit #8: Move Your Body!

The role of exercise. Do naturally thin people enjoy exercise more than chronic dieters? Not likely, many don't believe in exercising. They boast that they are the same weight as they were in college yet don't need to exercise. So it makes you wonder is it their metabolism? How can they stay slim without exercising? It is mainly because they move, naturally thin people move their bodies a lot more than the average person. They have "active" lifestyles. They walk more, take the stairs when given an option and generally move at a faster pace. If you watch a naturally thin person, they don't sit still very long. Studies show that lifestyle movement counts as exercise. Gardening, walking the dog, chasing the kids or grandkids, climbing stairs, just about any activity that gets your heart rate up.

Making time to move your body is essential for a healthy lifestyle. I recommend you begin with purchasing a pedometer. They are inexpensive and highly effective. Start the first few days with a baseline to see how many steps you take. Then make it your goal to take more steps the next day. Each day make it a goal to exceed the prior day. Naturally thin people actually take thousands of steps more than an overweight person. So this will take time to condition your body to consistently move more on a daily basis. By the time this happens you will have reduced your body fat, toned your muscles and more than likely be wearing a smaller size.

If you are ready to add exercise to your routine and don't know where to begin, start with walking. It is an excellent form of exercise. Begin with 20 minutes but strive for 40 when you feel strong. Exercising for 40 minutes will not only strengthen your heart but will begin to burn long chain fatty deposits. A rule is exercise 3 times per week for 30 minutes to strengthen your heart and 4 times per week for 40 minutes to burn fat.

When you are acclimated to walking and want to see more results, then I recommend working out with weights. I have seen tremendous results using a short and simple weight routine. Start with a basic routine and dumbbells. There are many versions in hundreds of books. Some are sitting on your bookshelf right now.

Make time to exercise, find something that is fun for you like riding your bike, walking, dancing – anything. Just move your body! People often ask me if they should exercise before or after they eat. There are many opinions about this. My personal goal is to burn fat so I like to work out first thing in the morning on an empty stomach. Your body wants to burn fuel and if you feed it right before you exercise, it will burn the sugar and calories from the meal.

When possible, exercise before eating (1 to 2 hours) then your body will have to burn the stored fuel, which is either a reservoir of carbs or stored fat. If that is too difficult or you would prefer to workout after dinner, wait a few minutes and then go for it. The best approach is one that works for you. Trust your intuition and move your body. Either way you are accomplishing your goal of turning your body into a fat burning machine!

Remember nobody says, "Gosh I wish I didn't exercise, I am in such good shape, what was I thinking?" They say, "I don't always feel like it but it sure is worth it." So call a friend and go for a walk, you'll be glad you did! A couple of my neighbors and I workout every weekday together. There are mornings I really am tired (5:30 am), but I think about them waiting for me and I drag myself out of bed. You really have to find something to do that is fun.

I have two favorite workouts. For cardio, I find kickboxing to be a great workout. My friends and I also love Turbo Jam™ by BeachBody; it is a fun, effective and available on DVD! Chalene Johnson is the creator and she is very motivating. I also have found weight training to be very effective. My all time favorite routine is in Montel Williams and Wini Linguvic's book "Body Change." It has an excellent program that is easy to follow. If you follow it for 21 days, you will see a difference in your body. It will tone you from head to toe.

That is my workout routine, cardio 3-5 times per week with Chalene and weight training 3 times per week with Montel and Wini. I do it all from home, either mine or my friends. My body fat is down to 21% and I feel better in my forties than when I was in my twenties. I don't own a treadmill or any machines, just a DVD player, dumbbells and a big ball.

Your Assignment

Find an exercise buddy and move, move, move!

Habit #9: Stay on Track, the 80/20 Rule.

When most people start a weight loss program they jump right in and make a lot of changes all at once. They say, "I will start working out everyday; I am giving up all carbs, caffeine, and no more snacking in between meals."

What happens next? Within one week they will have pulled a muscle and can't work out. They will be craving carbs with an intense hunger they never felt before. They will have had migraines from caffeine withdrawal and they will be snacking on cookies.

Do I sound skeptical? As a weight loss coach, I have seen thousands of people do this. Weight management is a lifestyle, not an event. You have to design a life that supports a healthy body. This takes time, maybe even years to cultivate.

We are accustomed to instant gratification and we are fortunate enough to live in society that renders results quickly in so many ways. We can walk up to a machine and with a swipe of a plastic card have cash in seconds. We can walk into the world's best grocery store – Wegmans (in Rochester, NY) and have a healthy gourmet meal ready to serve to our family. We are blessed this is a fact. But when it comes to our weight, we still have to do it the old fashion way. It takes time to lose weight. If we try to make a 180-degree shift from day one, it will take even longer.

This is because it will be difficult for you to sustain a change that is too painful or inconvenient. You are far better off making a small change and integrating it into your life, then moving on to another small change and integrating that one. I always tell my clients I am not asking you to make a 180-degree shift, only a five- degree shift. A plane that is only three degrees off course can arrive in a completely different country than its intended destination. So you can make a small shift and if you keep it consistent over time, you will make significant progress.

Naturally thin people don't obsess on food, they just move on. They know they will eat better later to make up for the "indulgence". If you feel you are struggling, then maybe you are doing too much, too fast. Make a small shift. Don't worry about getting off course. As long as you are on course more than you are off, you will be fine over the long run. Most airplanes are off course for most of the trip.

They have to continually redirect to reach their desired destination. The same is true with your weight management: as long as you on track more than off, you are making progress and over time you will arrive at your destination. So don't be so hard on yourself, decide what small shift you are able to make today that you know will add up over time. It took me a year to lose 30 pounds, but I thought, "Hey next year at this time I will be looking good."

Here are some small (5 degree) shifts that make a big difference over time. Pick one:

- Replace breakfast with a protein drink.

- Don't eat after 7:00 pm.

- Have a balance of protein and carbs when you eat.

- Avoid white flour.

- Avoid white sugar.

- Don't drink soda pop.

- Snack on veggies.

- Go for a walk four times a week.

Summary and Suggestions for the 9 Habits

Imagine what would happen if you applied just one of these for an entire year!

1. Take time each day to imagine yourself healthy and fit. Post a picture or photo of either yourself or someone whom you admire. It needs to be a flattering image, not of what you don't want; look at it often with excitement. This sounds a little self-absorbed, but it works. Your unconscious mind needs direction, a positive image to manifest. You will go in the direction of your most dominant thought. Become curious: ask yourself, "What would it be like to live in this body?" Naturally thin people imagine themselves looking good.

2. Develop a phrase that supports your goal. Make it simple and say it as if it were true. Think thoughts like, "Nothing tastes as good as a healthy, fit body feels." These types of thoughts will rewire your brain for success.

3. Stop dieting and eat food that you enjoy. Chew slowly, take your time, and be fully present. Savor your food. It takes up to 20 minutes for your brain to register that your stomach is satisfied. Watch a thin person when they eat, they take a few bites then they put down their fork and talk or just take a rest. While everyone else at the table has cleaned their plate, the naturally thin person has eaten only half of their serving.

4. Don't over eat. Eat only when you are physically hungry and stop when the hunger goes away. Listen to your body. Use the scale from 1-10: one is famished, ten is stuffed. Don't wait until you are too hungry. Eat when you are at a two, and stop when you are satisfied, a five. Basically, don't finish what you start. You will lose weight without deprivation.

5. Properly combine proteins, carbs and fats to assist your body in digestion and burning of fat. Eat foods that maximize your energy not deplete you of it. Become an expert of your body. Pay attention to what works for you. Then respect your body's needs. Read: "Avoid an Insulin Response". It will help you to accomplish this.

6. Move your body. Take in fewer calories than you burn. Eat the majority of your food during the day as opposed to evening. Since your body is burning the bulk of calories throughout the day, avoid eating at night. At night your body needs energy to replenish itself, not digest food.

7. Drink plenty of water. This will flush out toxins and broken down fatty deposits. When you lose weight, it doesn't just evaporate into thin air, you must eliminate it from your body. Drink at least eight glasses of water daily to effectively facilitate this process.

8. Move your body. Studies show that naturally thin people move around more than overweight people do. Lifestyle movement adds up quickly, find ways to move your body. It feels great and speeds up your metabolism which will burn more calories.

9. Follow the 80:20 rule. As long as you are following this 80% of the time, you are doing great! "All-or-nothing" is virtually impossible; when you fail it will discourage you and cause you to give up. Never give up, this is a lifestyle change, not an event. Naturally thin people eat a cookie and forget about it. They don't use it as an excuse to overeat.

Avoid an Insulin Response

Having worked with thousands of people, I have seen a common similarity that can be attributed to the reason 70% of my clients seem to gain weight so easily and struggle to take it off.

A big cause is due to them being insulin resistant. What this means is that their bodies react to the "sugar" in foods in such a way that they require excessive amounts of insulin to manage their blood sugar. When this dynamic occurs we call it an insulin response.

An insulin response (IR) is this: when you consume food the sugar within that food (also known as glucose) elevates your blood sugar – your body produces insulin to digest/reduce the glucose levels in your bloodstream. The more resistant you are, the more insulin needs to be produced. Once the proper amount of insulin is released then your blood sugar returns to a healthy range.

A person who is not resistant will be able to consume the same foods and may even provoke an IR but their body will produce minimal amounts of insulin to stabilize their blood sugar. It will quickly return to a normal range without dropping too low. That is the way it is supposed to happen for a healthy body that is not resistant to insulin. In time however if they have caused an IR too many times, then their body will little by little require more insulin to manage their blood sugar. Eventually they too will become insulin resistant and not understand why they can't eat the same foods they always have in the past.

Here is an example of an IR: if you eat a banana with a glass of orange juice for breakfast, it has a very high fructose content (sugar from fruit). The amount of sugar will be released into your bloodstream quickly and in a large amount. If you are a healthy person who isn't insulin resistant, your body may still experience IR except your body can manage it effectively.

Let's assume (these numbers are not fact), to accomplish this, your body needs to produce one part insulin to manage 5 parts sugar and your blood sugar is restored to normal. You will be able to eat this way with little weight gain or health risk.

But if you are insulin resistant, your body reacts differently to sugar, releasing too much glucose (sugar), too quickly into your bloodstream. This will spike your blood sugar producing an IR just like the first example except two things will occur that are different. One being that the insulin released will not manage your sugar level effectively thus requiring more insulin and second being that when it finally does, your blood sugar will drop too low. Let's look at both areas:

The first problem is that when your body releases one part of insulin to manage the (5 parts), sugar, **nothing happens,** so it needs to release more insulin until the blood sugar is managed. It may have to double that amount (because your body is "resistant" to the insulin), before the blood sugar returns to normal. (Again I am not stating actual numbers just making a point). In either case this is too much insulin for the body and is not a sign of a healthy balanced body.

Why is consistently releasing insulin a problem? Because this is a pre-diabetic state, it is only a matter of time and you will develop diabetes. If this is you then you have a reason for concern. The good news is that you have the information you need in this book to avoid causing further damage. If you are diabetic then you are playing with fire, you must manage your blood sugar levels now to restore your body to health. I have witnessed clients who have been taken off of their medication (by their doctors) because they have successfully managed insulin levels.

The second problem is that if someone is insulin resistant then the body may react to the excess amount of insulin by dropping the blood sugar, too low and below normal. When the blood sugar dips too low people become light headed, dizzy and experience cravings for sugar all over again. This is a natural way for the body to try to stabilize the blood sugar to normal. So they eat something like toast or drink a glass of juice to get the blood sugar up again. It will work, they will feel better for a short time until the blood sugar drops again, only to repeat the pattern, this cycle continues repeatedly throughout the day.

This roller coaster wave of blood sugar and insulin (IR) will set the foundation for a number of physical problems that are preventable, including weight gain. You do not want your diet to elevate insulin levels all day long. It will eventually reduce the quality of your health.

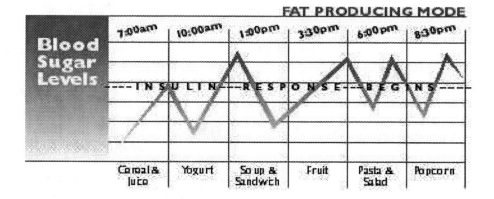

* From Mind Over Platter® Food Journal 2003

Frequent elevated insulin levels causes excess insulin in the body. When this hormone is out of balance you will encourage a host of problems:

- Your body to store fat, causing you to gain weight without overeating.

- Your kidneys to store sodium, who needs to retain more water?

- Your blood pressure can increase.

- Your liver to produce cholesterol.

- Your arteries to form plaque.

- Inflammation in your body, aggravating arthritis and joint pain.

One way to avoid this cycle is to avoid an IR. You can accomplish this easily by reducing the amount of starchy carbohydrates you consume and properly combining them with other foods. I call starchy carbohydrates impact carbs. The sugars in these carbs impact your blood sugar causing an IR. The bottom line is balance. You must balance your food intake to not overload the amount of sugar entering into the bloodstream at any given time. How do you do this? You must properly combine your food.

If you combine protein, fat, and carbohydrates properly then the protein and fat will slow down the blood sugar from rising too high. When eating carbohydrates, your best choices are fibrous foods. Which have a high water content as well as fiber including fruit. Eat plenty of salads and vegetables. The carbohydrates you will want to reduce are the impact carbs: the ones with white flour and sugar (breads, pasta, cereals, and sweets). I also consider white rice, potatoes, corn, peas, beets and fruits as impact carbs. Again it is the sugar content in the food that causes it to spike your blood sugar.

If you experience IRs and want to lose weight, your success depends on your ability to keep your protein intake equal to, or higher than impact carbs. This will allow you to burn fat rather than store fat. You need to do this each time you eat. If you are eating 10 grams of impact carbs, balance it with 20 grams of protein. It is that simple.

This doesn't include salads and most vegetables, they have little impact on your blood sugar. Only count the impact carb (food) grams and counter it with protein grams.

This is an over-simplified explanation of a complex physical reaction. Keep in mind that the main focus of this program is to eat food in moderation. Balance is key. Proper mixing of protein intake with glucose (sugar), intake changes the way the meal is processed. It can greatly reduce even eliminate IR. As long as you eat when you are physically hungry and stop the moment you're satisfied, you will lose weight. This practice has helped many people lose weight and keep it off. Let's take a look at another dynamic that is occurring within your body concerning impact carbs.

How to eat your cake and be thin too:

The body's fuel of choice is glucose, otherwise known as sugar. So when you consume a high impact carb meal (a plate of pasta and garlic bread) your body breaks that down into macronutrients: carbohydrates, fat and a small amount of protein. Perhaps your body only needs 25 % of the sugar from those carbs for energy. It will take the rest (glucose AKA sugar AKA impact carb) and store it in a reserve for later as fuel. But let's say you want a snack a couple of hours later, and you have some peanut butter and crackers, (impact carb, fat and protein) your body is still running on the pasta (glucose) fuel, so it will only need 15% of the glucose for the rest of the day. It stores the excess glucose for fuel for later.

Where does all of the stored fuel go if you don't burn it? Well first it is immediately stored within your muscles for fuel for the day. It continues to stock pile this fuel for about 24 hours assuming you are going to exert yourself and need the fuel to energize your body. I call this short-term parking. There are only so many spaces available in short term parking and every 24 hours it will empty out the parking lot and make room for the current days needs. If the fuel isn't used within that timeframe then the body has an efficient process; it transforms the fuel into fat and stores it in long-term parking. This is fuel for future use, not immediate energy.

Now let me clarify that your body is converting the fuel into fat and stores it within your fatty deposits. You have a certain number of fatty deposits in long-term parking, they will never leave. But they can shrink or expand to accommodate your parking needs. Each fatty deposit can shrink to the size of a grain of rice (actually smaller than that) and expand to the size of a baseball. So you will never run out of long-term parking. Where is long term parking physically located? You guessed it, on your hips, your belly and your thighs.

I should mention briefly, this doesn't seem to be a problem for people who are athletic or physically active. They burn their energy while it is in short-term parking and it never moves into long-term parking. If you are very active, in terms of exercise, and work out frequently, then you need the impact carbs for energy and performance enhancement.

For the rest of us who are gaining weight instead of losing on a low fat, high carb diet this is mainly why. We are taking in more fuel than we are burning from impact carbohydrates. Now here is the interesting part, protein with fat is not a preferred source of fuel for the body so it has a completely different chemical reaction than the impact carb. Protein will create a thermogenesis in your body by speeding up the metabolism. Your body ignores (so to speak) the calories from the protein and fat and seeks its fuel from glucose (impact carb calories) to burn. First it will utilize this from the food you are eating at each meal. Once that is depleted it will go to short-term parking. After that is depleted, it will go to long-term parking.

In other words if you are monitoring impact carbs and balancing them with protein and fat, your body will run out of it's preferred fuel source quickly. It will then go to the muscle storage (short-term parking). After a couple of days of this it will run out of fuel from short term parking and then go into the fuel stored in the long term parking lot. This is when it will finally burn fat from your hips, belly and thighs.

This can be a beautiful thing but first you have to find the best balance of protein and impact carbs for your body to reach this point. You could literally turn your body into a fat burning machine by properly balancing your food intake.

Be sure to check with your health care provider prior to changing your eating plan. Of course drink plenty of water, take a good multivitamin – and exercise.

Once you have reached your goal you can change that ratio of protein to impact carb, it is different for each person. Pay attention to your body.

PIC a Ratio *grams of Protein to grams of Impact Carbs*

As I stated earlier, I have followed a 2:1 ratio for years and it works for me. I eat two grams of protein to every one gram of impact carbs. I eat all of the vegetables I like and only monitor the carbs from bread, pasta, rice, potatoes, sugar, fruit, corn, peas and all sweets. I recommend you use a food journal to find your proper ratio and create a balance that works for you.

It is a matter of cracking your own fat burning code. The 2:1 ratio will work for a wide range of people. If you are eating 20 grams of protein then balance it with 10 grams of impact carbs. It will kick-start your metabolism. My Carb Addict Carla clients do very well with this ratio.

Many people can actually vary it, but as I said it requires time and testing to discover your balance. If you want to burn through short-term parking and burn up the spaces in long-term parking then try the 2:1 ratio. It is easy to follow, simple to remember. Then once you reach your goal, you can adjust the ratio and see what works for you to keep you within your ideal weight range.

If you are fortunate, and have a good metabolism, you might find you can consume a balance of 20 grams of protein and 30 grams of impact carbs and lose weight. I call this the 1:1.5 Ratio, Low Fat Laura usually does well with this ratio, because they are not typically insulin resistant.

Then we have the 1:1 Ratio, 20 grams of protein to 20 grams of carbs. This often works for Fast Pace Freddy because they are consuming two - three times that amount per meal. It might even work for Over Eating Oscar, depending on what provokes an IR for them

By using your food journal, you will be able to track this information for future reference and guidance.

There are a number of books written on this topic and you might want to further research it. My favorites include: "The Metabolic Plan", by Stephen Cherniske. "The Zone" by Barry Sears and "The South Beach Diet" by Arthur Agatston.

They are all excellent references with the same core concept. I encourage you to understand and follow the concept not the latest trend. Because the vast majority of my clients experiences an IR and like the 2:1 Ratio, I am going to focus on it for the remainder of this chapter.

Please consult with your health care provider. I am sharing with you my experience and insight but I am not a doctor and couldn't sleep at night blindly giving you advice. I am providing you with information that I am confident in and is accurate and up to date. It has held true for me and my clients. I believe we should each take responsibility for our own health and be as informed as possible. Especially about our bodies, and our own personal insight is unique to each of us. What works for one person may not for another, so get to know your body and your health.

What I do know is that white flour and white sugar have no need to be in your life and I won't feel guilty asking you to reduce even eliminate them from your eating plan.

I encourage you over the next few days to observe how your body responds to reducing or even eliminating white flour and sugar from your daily intake. As you have heard me say before it is an addictive drug and will cause your blood sugar to sky rocket only to crash within a couple of hours. This recreates the sugar/starch craving and causes "killer" cravings and an intense hunger. The result is that you eat more of what your body is reacting to. I am serious when I say it is an addiction – if not for everyone, at least for me as well as many of my clients.

If you notice you feel better with a low sugar/flour meal plan, with an increase of energy and weight loss, then it is probably true for you as well. This is something you are going to have to accept as a reality in life. It may be a bitter pill to swallow. But the sooner you face the truth the faster you can take back control over food and your weight. To this day, if I eat more than a couple of pieces of fruit or whole grain bread, my cravings increase, appetite is out of control and my weight will consistently climb.

It isn't fair but it is life. I have come to look at it as if I were upset because I have brown eyes. I never asked for brown eyes, I was just born with them, would I rather have Linda Carters blue eyes? Yes, but I have brown eyes. There are just some things in life you can't change and have to make the best of, and not having a high tolerance for impact carbs may be one of them.

Again your ratio could be different than mine. A 2:1 ratio works for a large number of people. Get to know your body and its limits; then respect it. Use your food journal to assist you. Don't spend too much time in denial, it will only lead you to gaining weight and a lot of frustration. So face reality, talk to your team and find a belief system that supports what is in your best interest.

I am in this with you. We will be healthier in the long run. You really can enjoy a healthier lifestyle eating this way.

What will you eat?

Breakfast is easy, an omelet with veggies and cheese, or cottage cheese with fresh fruit, or a protein drink. One of my favorites is whipped cottage cheese with raspberry low carb yogurt and fresh berries all mixed together, it is a real treat. If you are really hungry have some leftovers from last night's dinner.

Lunch is equally easy – a salad with grilled chicken, or tuna salad, or turkey breast. Dress your salad with balsamic vinegar and olive oil and load it up with olives, cucumbers, tomatoes and avocado. Another delicious meal is a low carb whole grain wrap. I have these with chicken salad, or roasted chicken breast, or beef strips. They are yummy. You will be hooked.

Dinner is the easiest, grill meat (steak, salmon, chicken, etc), and veggies, mash some cauliflower (add butter and cheddar cheese) and don't forget your salad on the side. Stir-fry is always an option. You can have shrimp, beef or chicken. And throw in some cashews with your favorite sauce. The possibilities are endless.

Snack (if you feel hungry) on peanuts, raw almonds, peanut butter and celery, string cheese, veggies and dip, hard boiled eggs, soy chips, salsa, sugar free Jell-O or pudding.

Listed on the next two pages are charts to help you better understanding this concept.

The first is a menu plan demonstrating the 2:1 PIC ratio. It is only counting Impact Carb foods, not carbs from vegetables.

The second is a grouping of foods and their macronutrient break down. You are basically picking food from each category. Eat in moderation, I don't believe in measuring food, just keep an eye on the Impact Carb and keep your fat portion to a serving size. A meal or snack consists of a protein, vegetables, an Impact Carb and a fat source.

Nuts and dairy are listed in the Fat grouping but do not have Impact Carbs, so you can technically have them as a snack alone and they won't provoke an Insulin Response. I am partial to nuts and snack on them often. But the calories can add up quickly so monitor them. Dairy I love as well, but can be too much fat if consumed consistently in high volumes. Keep an eye on your cholesterol and triglycerides to be sure your diet is not only keeping your weight down but healthy as well. My cholesterol was higher when I was a vegetarian than it is now. I firmly believe you are the best expert in your body, get to know it well.

Meal:	Protein : Impact Carb

Breakfast:

3-egg omelet with steamed broccoli, 2 oz. Cheddar cheese,

1 slice of rye toast, butter, ¼ apple — 30 : 15

3/4 c. cottage cheese, 1 c. fresh strawberries — 21 : 10

Spinach frittata with mushrooms, tomatoes, Feta cheese

(no potatoes), 1 slice of whole grain toast, buttered — 30 : 15

Lunch:

Caesar salad (no croutons), with 4 oz. chicken — 25 : 12

Open face sandwich with 1 slice of bread, 4 oz. grilled meat,

cheese, slices of tomato, salad with dressing, melon — 35 : 20

Brown bag: Tuna or lunch meat on low carb pita with cheese,

cucumber slices with dip, raw almonds, ½ peach — 35 : 20

Dinner:

Broiled salmon with lemon butter, broccoli, 1/2 c. wild rice,

salad with pecans and Italian dressing — 36 : 20

Grilled chicken, 1/2 baked potato with sour cream, spinach

salad with bacon dressing — 35 : 20

6 oz. Steak, mushrooms, salad with oil and vinegar dressing,

1 multi grain roll with butter — 42 : 21

Snacks:

1/2 apple (sliced) with 3 oz. sharp Cheddar cheese — 18 : 10

Soy chips with fresh ground peanut butter — 18 : 12

Veggies and dip mixed with 1/2 c. Tofu — 10 : 5

Low carbohydrate Protein Shake — 15 : 5

Pick a food from each of the 4 categories to create a fat burning meal:

#1 **Protein: 4-6 oz** **(7 grams protein / ounce)**	#2 **Vegetables:** **(don't count carbs from)**	#3 **Fats/ Dairy/Nuts** **Fat:**
Whole Chicken & Breast	Broccoli	**(fat, 0 protein)**
Turkey Ground & Legs	Asparagus	Extra Virgin Olive Oil
Duck, Cornish Hen	Cauliflower	Black Olives
Fresh Tuna Steak	Bamboo Shoots	Greek Olives
Salmon Fillets	Peppers (red & green) Summer Squash	Real Mayonnaise
Lobster Whole & Tails	Cherry Tomato	Real Butter
Shrimp (frozen & fresh)	Brussels Sprouts	Cream Cheese
Fish (all types)	Crisp Sauerkraut	Sour Cream
Steak, Sirloin, Strip, etc	Avocados	**Dairy**
Beef (ground)	Butternut Squash	**(fat, 7 grams protein/oz)**
Baked Ham	Acorn Squash	Cottage Cheese
Pork, tenderloin, chops, etc.	Eggplant	Ricotta Cheese
Eggs and Egg Beaters	Cabbage	Feta Cheese
Tofu, fresh	Zucchini	Cheddar Cheese
Lean Deli Meat:	Snow Peas Green Beans	Swiss Cheese
Turkey, Chicken Breast, Ham, Roast Beef	Celery	Munster Cheese
Tuna Fish (canned)	Artichokes Lettuce All Varieties	Provolone Cheese
Protein Shake: Soy & Whey	Spinach	Mozzarella Cheese
Turkey Bacon	Cucumbers	Monterey Jack Cheese
	Swiss Chard	Yogurt (no sugar added)
#4 Impact Carbs:	Mushrooms	Mascarpone Cheese
(a 15-20 gram serving)	Alpha Sprouts	Real Whipped Cream
Soy Chips	Cabbage	**Nuts & Seeds** **(fat, 8 protein/serving)**
Long Grain Brown Rice	Jalapenos	Raw Almonds
Whole Grain / Rye Bread	**Misc (free foods):** Vinegar	Cashews
Whole Wheat Pasta	Fresh Herbs / Spices	Dry Roasted Peanuts
Low Carb Wraps	Mustard / Horseradish	Pecans
Potatoes	Tabasco / Hot Sauce	Walnuts
Slow Cooked Oatmeal	Sugar Free Beverages	Macadamia Nuts
Barley, Lentils, Beans (dry)	Sugar Free Jello	Brazilian Nuts
Sugar Free Pudding		Pumpkin Seeds
All Fruits		Sunflower Seeds
All Sweets		Peanut Butter

Insulin Response Levels and Sugar:

What if I told you that you could increase your energy and reduce your cravings for sweets? Would you be interested in what I have to say? I can tell you what to do, but I don't want you to take my word for it, I want you to see for yourself.

I invite you to be part of an experiment. **Decide to be sugar free for seven days.** Eat only foods that won't convert into sugar rapidly in the bloodstream. Notice how you feel cutting out the sugar and flour products for just seven days.

I am betting you will feel more energy, optimistic and those sugar cravings will diminish.

An effective way to reduce sugar is to avoid foods that are high on the "Table of Insulin Response". The chart ranks food based on how quickly the glucose (sugar) within the food converts to sugar in your bloodstream. It basically is telling you how the food will impact your blood sugar. The higher the ranking the higher the impact.

- ➢ Foods that rank under 20 are in a no impact zone.
- ➢ Under 39 are in the low impact zone.
- ➢ Under 59 are in a moderate impact zone.
- ➢ Foods between 59-70 will have an impact on your blood sugar and can easily cause an Insulin Response. You might be able to manage it provided you balance the meal with a no impact food.
- ➢ Above 70 you are in the high impact carb zone.

* When counting impact carbs grams, count the ones that rank above 30 on the chart. Don't calculate the ones below 29 in your daily intake.

Table of Insulin Response

The higher the number the faster the food converts into glucose, causing blood sugar to rise rapidly. This can provoke an insulin response. The lower the number the slower the conversion. Your goal is to avoid an insulin response. Pick foods & combine foods that rate below 59.

Millet, Broad Beans, Dates, Potato, Cornflakes	101-140
Parsnips, Glucose, Popcorn, Rice Cakes, Honey, Dates	
Cereals: Cheerios, Total, Rice Krispies, Cream of Wheat	101-115
Pretzels, Watermelon, Puffed Wheat, Fat Free Cookies	
Donuts, White Bagels, Waffles, White Bread, Pancakes	
Glucose, Melba Toast, Grapenuts, Shredded Wheat,	90-100
Cream of Wheat, Cornmeal, Wheat Bread, Raisins	
Pineapple, Sucrose, Beets, Mueseli, Fat Free Ice Cream	
Corn Chips, Carrots, Yogurt w/ Fruit, Frozen Fat Free Yogurt	
White Rice, Instant Oatmeal, Apricots, Split Pea Soup	80 - 89
Potato Chips, Oat Bran, Banana, Cookies	
Pumpernickel Bread, Special K, Brown Rice, Corn	70 - 79
Orange Juice, Sweet Potato, Baked Beans, All Bran	
Mango, Papaya, Canned Beans, Buckwheat, Yams	
Grapes, Orange, Enriched Pasta, Peas, Lactose, Rye	60 - 69
Yogurt (artificially sweetened), Ice Cream, Beans (can)	
Pear, Plum, Apple Juice, Pinto & Black-Eyed Beans	50 - 59
Custard, Plain Yogurt, Wheat Pasta, Chick Peas	
Dried Peas & Beans, Skim Milk, Lima Beans, Rye Crisps	40 - 49
Old Fashion Rolled Oats, Protein Pasta, Lentils, Apples, Soy Chips	
Barley, Whole Milk, Grapefruit, Cherries, Fructose	30 - 39
Green Apple, Peach, Rice Bran, Tomatoes, Berries, Peanut Butter	
Soy Beans, Cauliflower, Artichoke, Asparagus, Sprouts	20 - 29
Broccoli, Most Raw Vegetables, (vegetables not listed above rank here)	
All Meat, Fish, Seafood, Cheese, Nuts	under 20

* This chart is based on the Glycemic Index

Keep a record of the foods you eat in your food journal and see how you feel in seven days. Rate each day based on your energy level 1-100%. Are you running on 50%, what is typical for you, what is productive for you?

When I eat a veggie omelet for breakfast and workout in the morning I feel like I am at 90%, I get a lot done. When I eat a donut and skip the workout, I am at 70% for about an hour then crash to 30%; I drag myself through the morning. I have noticed a major difference, when I stop to pay attention.

Your Assignment:

- Commit to a week
- Write down what you eat in your food journal
- Rate how you feel
- Monitor your weight
- Share your insights with your team.

Road Blocks to Weight Loss

So far I have provided you with a lot of information as well as opportunities to successfully reprogram your mind to think like a naturally thin person. I have even shared with you ways of eating to help your body burn fat like a naturally thin person. In addition to all of these great resources, I still have clients who do everything right and yet don't lose weight. When this happens I look at a number of areas.

First are they clinging to limiting beliefs? Do they have something to gain from being overweight, is it protecting them in some way? Then I look at their self-talk. Are they giving their subconscious minds negative or conflicting messages? I look at their "comfort zone" and their needs and values, do they need to set some boundaries? And of course I look at their food journal to see what they are eating. Very often I find foods that are not creating a fat burning metabolism. Now if they are following my suggestions and not making progress I have learned to look at other areas that could be creating a road block.

A common one is the medications they are taking. This is out of my scope so I encourage them to work with a doctor and a nutritionist simultaneously, which has proven to be successful.

There are a number of reasons responsible for sluggish weight loss. I will share with you five common obstacles that have been the source of many of my clients' frustration. I will be briefly discussing this topic over the next five chapters.

These most common road blocks that I encounter include: food sensitivities, a need for supplements, a need for detoxification, stress and a hectic lifestyle.

Food Sensitivities

This is a commonly overlooked culprit to why many people do not lose weight. The have a sensitivity or even a mild allergy to certain foods. I consider Carb Addict Carla to be a good example of someone who is sensitive to white flour and white sugar. They crave food with white flour for example, then eat the food they crave and feel lousy afterwards. They notice they are bloated, gassy, and uncomfortable and to top it all off, they have gained a couple of pounds. This is overlooked because we think of hives as a sign of an allergy. But with food it can be mild and more importantly a subtle reaction.

The body reacts to the food it is sensitive to. This reaction includes bloating, gas, headaches, mood swings, increased heart rate, hyperactivity, inflammation of joints, water retention and an intense craving for the food.

How do you know if you are reacting to a certain food? One sign is that you will crave it, we are very often allergic to what we crave. When you eliminate if from your diet you will experience a "withdrawal" which results in the body craving the substance. Once you indulge in it the craving is satisfied for a short period of time, then it returns with more intensity. This is why alcoholics must abstain 100% to be successful. Their body doesn't metabolize alcohol in the same manner as a person who is not allergic, which is why it is considered an illness rather than a psychological addiction.

Physical addictions and / or reactions are not going to be resolved by thinking thin, they must be treated properly. Alcoholics benefit from a comprehensive program including detoxification and lifelong support, food sensitivity is not as drastic. There are varying degrees with foods ranging from a delayed reaction of water retention to noticeable inflammation of the joints (which will ache), to full blown hives and difficulty breathing.

The way to identify a food allergy or sensitivity is to monitor what you are eating. Keep a food journal and notice how you feel right after you eat, a few hours later as well as the next day. If you notice your heart is racing and you had a beverage with caffeine, then pay attention the next time you consume caffeine.

If your heart begins to beat faster, then you are probably sensitive to caffeine. If you are bloated, your feet are swollen and your eyes are puffy, ask yourself what did I just eat? What did I eat yesterday? Look for the pattern, if every time you eat Chinese you wake up with puffy eyes, then you have evidence that you are sensitive or allergic to something in the Chinese food.

Once you have noticed the pattern avoid the food for a series of days and see how you feel. I would recommend you avoid the offending food for at least 21 days. That allows it to detoxify from your body. Then only have a small amount occasionally, if your body reacts again, stay away from it for an extended period of time. It isn't that the food is directly harming your body, but the inflammation and water retention, headaches, etc are throwing your body out of balance. A balanced body loses weight easier, heals itself faster and will help you to feel more energy. Over a long period of time subjecting yourself to foods that are the cause of inflammation, joint pain, headaches, heart palpitations and weight gain will cause damage to your body.

Common foods that are the source of sensitivity or an allergy:

- Flour based (white or wheat are most common)

- Sugar (glucose, fructose, lactose, sucrose, watch them all)

- Sodium and MSG

- Food with dyes (especially red)

- Additives in food and beverages (sulfites, nitrates, etc)

- Wheat based products

- Corn and corn by products (like corn syrup)

- Yeast (includes brewers yeast)

- Dairy products including eggs

- Fish/Meat: especially shell fish or red meat

If you suspect a food sensitivity or allergy, you might want to be tested for foods and food allergies by a trained professional.

If you are curious about how your body reacts do the following assignment: Keep a log of the foods you are eating and notice how your body reacts to various categories of foods. Rank these reactions either positive or negative. Then rate foods that you are reacting to in subcategories that indicate toleration levels such as "sensitive", "intolerant", or "allergic" Here are some scenarios using common foods:

When you eat food with too much yeast or white flour and you feel bloated afterwards, you might call that sensitive but tolerant. You can continue to eat those foods but there will be a consequence from it. You might gain weight and feel tired but you could live a normal life consuming this food within moderation.

When you eat food with MSG, your joints swell and your face becomes puffy, your heart palpitates and you feel terrible as a result, label it less tolerant, since the symptoms show up so quickly. You can continue to eat that food but it will cause you a source of noticeable discomfort.

When you drink milk, you immediately feel nauseous and may even throw up and you have diarrhea, your body doesn't tolerate milk. You go out of your way to avoid milk or anything that tastes or smells like it, you are intolerant to milk.

When you eat peanuts you immediately break out in hives and have trouble breathing resulting in a trip to the emergency room, you are severely allergic to peanuts.

Rate foods on how your body reacts to them, sensitive to intolerant. Pay attention to this by isolating food groups and keeping a food journal with your observations.

Supplements and Weight Loss

When the body is nutritionally out of balance it will cause a host of problems, including the inability to maintain ideal weight. Restoring your body to good health helps it to balance itself and makes it much easier for the body to break down stored fat. You will not only feel better but you will lose weight faster when you are in balance. An ideal way to accomplish balance within the body is to supplement with herbs, vitamins, minerals and essential fatty acids.

Many of my clients are deficient in similar nutrients. Once we restore the system to balance they seem to lose weight. I offer a nutrient analysis to my clients which signal out where they are deficient as well as if they are overstressing their liver, kidneys, adrenals, etc. If you haven't had a nutrient assessment done you might want to consider it. Speak to your nutritionist about having one done or you can fill out a form online. Many companies offer them including MindOverPlatter.com. It will reveal what supplements you need if any. Since most people consume a diet that is lacking proper nutrition their bodies are "running on empty" as far as nutrients go.

Food is a source of fuel, yet people eat mainly for comfort, and on the run. Healthy fuel sources are fresh foods, lean protein, nuts, salads, whole grains, legumes (not from a can), rich-deep colored fruits and vegetables. If your body is insulin-resistant then you will be avoiding the foods that cause your blood sugar to sky rocket. Those foods would include some fruits, breads, etc. Because few people are fueling their bodies adequately, nutritional supplements can make a difference in your energy level as well as rate of weight loss.

Another reason people don't lose weight and have more belly fat can be due to stress and the production of cortisol. This hormone can cause intense hunger and cause you to gain weight. There has been a lot of hype on this topic, I would prefer you avoid the latest tend and look at the source of the problem. One being stress due to the busyness of a fast paced life style that is not in balance. Second is a need for supplements to support your adrenal glands, which are overworked due to your fast paced lifestyle.

Once you have determined what you need and what system is being stressed then you need to repair, restore and rebuild the body. The way I like to accomplish this is with herbs and supplements. I am a big fan of herbs especially Chinese blends. Chinese medicine has been around for thousands of years and is focused on keeping the body healthy, not fixing it when it is broken. It also is based on the source of the problem rather than the symptom. What I have discovered about herbs is that when you take them you will have a number of side benefits, unlike drugs where you will experience a number of side effects. I have a free chart included on MindOverPlatter.com if you are interested in further recommendations about supplements. For now here is a list of my favorite supplements that are proven to be useful for weight loss.

Hoodia Formula: a stimulate free appetite suppressant.

Nature's Cortisol: to counteract the over production of cortisol.

Adrenal Support: will feed your adrenal glands and help you to relax.

Food Enzymes: to help your body digest protein, fats carbohydrates.

CLA: Essential Fatty Acids, burns fat and sustains muscle mass.

Fat Grabbers: absorbs and eliminates excess fat in your diet.

Calcium Magnesium: proven to assist in weight loss.

NutriCalm: rich in B complex vitamins with will combat stress.

Chinese Mood Elevator: to lift your spirits and stabilize your mood.

Carbo Grabbers: to intercept absorption of calories from impact carbs.

Vital Wave: a complete multi-vitamin with minerals in liquid form.

Dieter's Cleanse: a cleansing program that promotes detoxification.

Nature's Three: high fiber supplement that I drink daily.

For information visit: http://www.mynsp.com/smith25/index.aspx

Detoxify Your Body

Cleansing

I know this is not a topic that is discussed in most weight loss books, but I have been a student of natural health my whole life. The fact that this is rarely discussed is plain and simply irresponsible. It is a cornerstone of health.

Cleansing your system is important. Because even if you are eating healthy and taking the right supplements they may not be doing your body any good if it is toxic. Vitamins and minerals need to be assimilated by your body, if your colon is clogged or caked with toxins or fecal matter it will not absorb the supplements or nutrients.

What will a cleansing do? There are a number of benefits first, it will clean out the accumulation of the fecal matter that has been adhering to the intestinal walls. This may have been accumulating for years and is toxic matter. You can have 5-20 pounds of fecal matter build up. One thing I like about a cleanse is how noticeably flatter your abdominal area gets from it. You can see the difference because you won't have that bloated feeling.

Second, a cleanse will detoxify your liver and other organs. Your liver has to process food and nutrients for your body to run efficiently. If you consume alcohol, drink coffee, smoke, or take any type of medication then your liver is exposed to toxins. It is working harder than it needs to just to process these toxins.

Third, a cleanse will eliminate parasites. I know this isn't a pleasant topic, but it is a fact of life. We are all exposed to parasites. If you have been out of the country, have pets or eat raw or rare meat (including sushi) there is a good chance you have encountered parasites. What very likely happens is that your parasites will feed off of the food you are eating and your body is not absorbing the nutrients in the food. Over time your body will break down, even though you are taking care of your self.

Forth: a cleanse will eliminate toxins that are stored in your fatty deposits. Your body protects your heart and organs from toxins by placing them within fatty deposits. The problem with this is your body holds on to the fat to keep your body safe from the toxins.

This is stubborn fat, once you cleanse and the toxins are eliminated the body releases the fat. I have seen many of my clients body fat go down after a cleanse.

The change in season is a good time to cleanse your system. When I say system I mean your intestines, colon, and liver. If you want to kick start your weight loss, then consider a cleansing.

As you can see I am a fan of cleansing, and on a regular basis, say, two-four times per year. I like to cleanse when the seasons change, or when I have abused my body. When I refer to "abused", for me that means too much alcohol, red meat, sushi, caffeine, processed foods or have taken medication. By the "worlds" standards, my diet is fine, by mine I am overwhelming my system.

To cleanse your system, you can fast. This is difficult to stick with but if you decide to try this, become educated in it first. I have done the Master Cleanse, it is a blend of distilled water, maple syrup, fresh lemon juice and cayenne pepper.

My favorite way to cleanse is with herbs. You are probably not surprised since I believe there is an herbal answer to any problem. My favorites:

Dieter's Cleanse: is a safe, simple, convenient cleansing program. It provides dietary fiber, supports the production of digestive enzymes and promotes detoxification.

Nature's Three: high fiber supplement that I drink daily.

Stress and Weight Loss

From my years of studying natural health and wellness, I consider the number one problem that will cause the most damage is stress. Stress causes headaches, backaches, high blood pressure, compromises your immune system and is a major factor in heart attacks. If all this wasn't enough, stress can cause you to gain weight.

If your stress levels are high and you are gaining weight consider a supplement to counterbalance your cortisol production. High levels of stress and chronic stimulation of the hormone cortisol will cause an increase in appetite, craving for carbs and weight gain.

Now if this isn't bad enough gaining weight (due to stress or overeating) will cause you to feel more stress. I know first hand, that when you are a stress eater and you gain weight, it only intensifies your stress. I am not suggesting that you can live a stress-free life, it is how your deal with stress that really matters. You can manage stress, it is your choice. Ask yourself, "What purpose does this feeling serve?" and "What has to happen right now so that I can feel harmony instead?"

Creating a healthy lifestyle is all about balance. Balance is not an accident, you will need to manage various aspects of your life to create balance. Don't wait until you are overwhelmed and exhausted before you take action to reduce stress. The body is like a robot, it is easily conditioned.

What you do consistently will be conditioned and become automatic. If you live with a certain amount of stress and don't address it, your body will react by becoming nervous more frequently and with little reason. Don't wait another day, manage stress today.

Thinking Thin Thought:

Repeat these words when you feel stressed. *"Stress is a choice and I choose peace instead. I am free of stress in this moment"*

Your Assignment:

Be proactive, decide that you will integrate some of the suggestions listed to counter or even reduce the stress in your life.

- Pray

- Meditate

- Write in your journal.

- Sleep 8 hours per night.

- Breath, take some nice long deep breaths.

- Exercise 3-5 times per week.

- Go for a walk.

- Spend time outside with nature, on the water, in a park.

- Avoid toxic people who try to control you, gossip, are needy, complain, or drain you in any way.

- Catch up on the details of life, fill your gas tank, keep your dentist appointments, and don't wait until the last minute.

- Read a good book.

- Take your supplements and medication.

- Eat healthy foods.

- Get involved in a hobby or activity that makes you smile.

- Delegate chores and tasks whenever possible.

- Listen to a meditation, visualization or self-hypnosis CD's.

- Practice the "Freedom Formula" (outlined in this book).

- Meet with your Weight Loss Support Team weekly and talk about what strategies are working for you.

Losing Weight While Managing a Busy Lifestyle

With the busy lifestyle most people live, making time for themselves is often low on the priority list. It has become a stressful time for many. In the midst of working, shopping, housecleaning, taking care of kids, pets, and parents, when do you find time to eat healthy? Also an increase in stress levels can often stimulate your appetite causing you to eat more than you realize.

One distinction I would point out concerns the difference between busy and hectic. I personally like to be busy and am probably one of the busiest people I know. But I avoid a hectic lifestyle. My personal boundary is in this area, I don't mind a busy day, but I do not tolerate a hectic one.

For me, busy is planned time, I have a lot to do, but have it scheduled so that I can manage it well and with little stress. A hectic schedule is often overlapping appointments, caused by outside influences. I do my best to avoid hectic, which is when I may need to say "no" to remain in harmony with my values. Now to someone else, my busy day may be hectic to them. So it is up to you to determine what you are comfortable with. Even with a busy life you must have a game plan for food.

Most people plan their vacations flawlessly but don't plan their meals. Living on pizza, doughnuts, and fast food for a few days per week could easily cause a 5- 25 pound weight gain. A poor diet will also deplete your body's energy and be the cause of mood swings.

You may have to delegate cooking and chores to manage eating healthy while keeping up a busy pace. This will require communicating with your family on what you need and expect from everyone. By doing this, you will be demonstrating to your family how to communicate your needs as well as showing them that it is okay to take care of yourself.

One of these needs will be time to unwind. Build "down time" into your day. A hot bath, time to read, prayer, and meditation will help you to clear your mind and experience more peace during this stressful time.

Here are helpful hints for making your busy life a healthy one:

☐ Plan ahead; make a list of your meals for the week. Just like you have a to-do list, have a meal list. Sit and write down your snack and meal plan for the entire week. Don't wait until you are hungry to think about this.

☐ Go grocery shopping on a full stomach, after you have eaten a healthy meal. Then shop and buy what is on your list.

☐ Keep a supply of fresh fruits and vegetables in the refrigerator. Stock up on nonperishable food in your cupboard, raw almonds, dry roasted peanuts, walnuts, albacore tuna, sugar free pudding, jello, and soda, in case you are hungry and aren't eating for a while.

☐ For kids, keep fresh fruit, natural granola bars, juice boxes, peanut butter, whole grain crackers, string cheese, and fitness water. Avoid buying them chips and snacks that even you might be tempted with.

☐ Keep bottled water, cut veggies, fruit, low-fat cheese, hard-boiled eggs and protein shakes in a cooler in your car. Then if you are in between stops you can have a healthy snack.

☐ Start the day off with a healthy breakfast that includes protein. This will stabilize your blood sugar and reduce cravings for sweets.

When Dining Out:

Have a game plan. I like to know in advance what I am going to order. This helps me to avoid temptation and ordering impulsively. In my mind I am thinking "those cheese fries look good" but my mouth says "I'll have the salad with grilled chicken, without the croutons." If I am really in the mood to indulge, I don't even look at the menu.

Here are examples of what to order while dining out:

- Chinese food: order your entree steamed with the sauce on the side.

- Italian: Chicken French with vegetables.

- Mexican: Salad with grilled chicken or a low carb quesadilla (to share).

- Chain Restaurant: Salad with grilled salmon or chicken, hold the croutons and bread.

- Greek: Shish kabob and a Greek salad.

- Steakhouse: A lean cut of steak, vegetables and a salad.

- Seafood: Anything that is broiled with vegetables and a salad.

- Breakfast: Any omelet loaded with vegetables, your favorite cheese and rye toast with butter on the side, hold the potatoes.

- Find places that serve salads with chicken or salmon, ask for dressing on the side.

- Have an appetizer as your meal or share an entrée, the portions are large enough.

- If you are ordering dessert, share it with a friend.

I think by now you are getting the idea, the pattern is simply protein, vegetables, and salad with a small serving of an impact carbohydrate.

In case you eat on the run often and tend to grab fast food, pick up menus from restaurants that offer "curb side pick up." Some of them will come out to your car and deliver food right to you.

Also watch your alcohol intake, the calories add up fast. If you do drink, develop a taste for dry red wine, at least it has healthy benefits (one glass). Avoid mixed drinks that are sweet.

Your Assignment:

➢ Make the distinction for yourself on what is busy and what is hectic.

➢ Establish guidelines that allow you to avoid living a hectic life and share this with your family.

➢ Share your guidelines with your Team.

➢ Hold each other accountable to follow through on guidelines.

The Freedom Formula

This formula is basic and it actually works! Exercise it daily. Repeating this cycle on a daily basis conditions your nervous system. This relaxing feeling should stimulate the parasympathetic nervous system, which is also triggered in a similar way after a hearty meal.

Your parasympathetic nervous system releases endorphins, which allows you to feel euphoric. The only difference is that you are satisfied and relaxed without using food.

First you need to practice by taking a deep relaxing breath, now hold it for a moment, then slowly exhale. I like to breathe in through my nose and exhale through my mouth. It conditions my mind and my body.

Repeat to yourself the word "re - lax". Break it up so that you are thinking "re" as you inhale and "lax" as you exhale.

Allow all of your awareness to focus on the space between breathing in and out, between "re" and "lax".

As you are breathing, imagine a warm white light relaxing you from the top of your head to the tips of your toes.

While you are feeling peaceful, breathing slowly, imagine yourself in your healthy body, say your power phrase and allow yourself to feel excited and optimistic.

Your Assignment

Condition the **Freedom Formula** daily.

1. Take a deep breath, thinking "re" – "lax", for a few cycles.

2. Imagine your ideal image, and repeat your power phrase.

3. Clench your left fist and take a look at it. Your stomach is about the same size. You only need a small portion of food to feel satisfied. If you are unsure cut your usual portion in half.

4. Eat what you really want. Make a healthy selection that is also tasty.

5. Truly enjoy your food, chew slowly. This will activate the enzymes in your salvia, which will help you to digest food easily and effortlessly.

6. Stop eating the moment you are satisfied (not full, a number 5). Remember: number 10 is stuffed. Take a deep breath, repeat to yourself "re" - "lax" cycle, feel this comfortable feeling.

7. Clench your left fist and look at it. Your stomach doesn't require a large portion of food. Push the plate away. When it comes to food develop the habit of not finishing what you start.

8. Feel proud of yourself, knowing that you control food and it does not control you!

9. Imagine how good you will look and feel once you have reached your goal. Repeat your power phrase and smile anticipating how great this will feel!

How Far Will a Change Go?

This has been a great journey of self discovery. Weight management is far more than counting calories. It is a lifestyle. I hope that you integrate the suggestions that we have been discussing here and with your team. Even if you apply one suggestion, it could literally change your life. You never know how far a change will go. Think about it, how far can a change really go? Let me tell you a story about Rhonda, she weighed 230 pounds with 50% body fat. Now Rhonda had a history of heart disease and diabetes, her mother had it as well as her grandmother. She decided to make one change and see what happened. Habit number one most appealed to her: Imaging herself healthy and fit. She would visualize herself in a healthy trim body every morning.

Rhonda is an active member of MindOverPlatter.com, so when she read that imagination is the language of the subconscious mind. It reinforced her decision to visualize herself weighing 150 pounds and feeling healthy. She also learned to supercharge her image with emotion to get excited about it. So for the fun of it she spent 2 minutes per day seeing herself in a healthy fit 150 pound body and let herself get excited about it. She saw herself at work and at parties looking good and feeling great.

On the days Rhonda visualized with emotion her ideal body, she would make healthier food choices mainly because she couldn't get that image out of her head. Then after work she would go for a walk because she had energy from not overeating during the day. She wasn't hungry after walking and didn't snack at night. When she woke up in the morning she felt more alert because she didn't have a sugar hangover from the night before. This morning ritual was actually fun for her because she was beginning to believe it would become a reality. And it did, about 18 months later Rhonda reached her goal!

One day at a holiday party Rhonda was wearing a very flattering outfit that honestly she felt like a million bucks in. She was beaming with energy. She was so excited about her life and people were complementing her daily. In addition to this Rhonda just received the results from her doctor's visit, she was at 25% body fat, her triglycerides and cholesterol was the lowest it a very long time! She was managing her sugar levels with her diet.

She was breaking a pattern that had been in her family for generations. Rhonda's life has changed, she started buying trendy clothes, enjoyed wearing some make-up and even decided to try a new hair style. Rhonda had known her hair stylist for years and they were becoming good friends. She found her stylist to be very supportive during her weight loss process and spoke openly about her discoveries. One day while at the beauty salon her stylist shares with Rhonda what an inspiration she has been to her. The stylist tells her that she had been living with an abusive partner and did not confine in anyone. She wished she had the inner strength to leave.

Seeing Rhonda's transformation make her wonder if she could duplicate similar results. She secretly began the ritual Rhonda spoke about of visualizing every morning, it was easy and Rhonda swore by it. Every morning she would see herself happy and confident, successfully supporting herself in her own peaceful and safe home, this would fill her with hope. This hope, in time began to motivate her, she realized she needed to ask for help and seek counseling. After a short time, the counselor helped her to build her self esteem. She started to feel more secure within her self and her confidence grew. Her new found confidence gave her the courage she needed to move out and not look back. Now the stylist seemed to be stronger, glowing with love and on the road to a happier life. It all started with a casual conversation.

Your life is touching so many others in a positive way. I believe God uses our lives to help others. What is the point of only helping ourselves? When we can use our insight and knowledge to help others find their path to peace and happiness then you are fulfilling God's purpose for you. You never know how far a change will go.

Your Assignment:

- ❖ Visualize with feeling your ideal body and your ideal life. Get excited about it, jump up and down, and listen to upbeat music.
- ❖ Make this one change and notice how far it will go.
- ❖ Share this image with supportive people.

You Have Come a Long Way Baby!

I would like to thank you for allowing me to be your guide through your weight loss journey. It is an honor to share this wonderful experience with you. I have used this information I'm sharing with you to not only lose weight, but keep it off. I have seen my clients lose 80 + pounds applying it. It really works.

You have come a long way. You've begun with aligning your inner truth by letting yourself experience self-love and acceptance. This is a peaceful and healing process in itself. Then you took the time to design an attainable outcome and set some realistic goals. You have developed a plan of action, which you have been following by using your food journal. You have learned the Nine Common Habits of Naturally Thin People.

By now you have been repeating your Power Phrase and visualizing your empowering ideal image daily. You have learned how important it is to eat when you are physically hungry and stop the moment that you are satisfied. You have practiced the Freedom Formula to condition your nervous system and now you can use it to easily experience peace and relaxation.

You understand how to avoid an Insulin Response (IR). You have insight into your eating patterns, having tracked it consistently. You have learned about your food triggers and you now have a plan of what to do rather than overeating.

You have learned about the power of your beliefs and added some empowering new members to your Committee.

You have many resources available to you. How can you not succeed? It is only a matter of time and you will not only reach your goal, you will exceed your expectations.

You have done a great deal of work. I am proud of you. You should feel proud of yourself. Only strong and motivated people will take the time to discover what they really need to do to manifest a healthy body. You are awesome. I am looking forward to hearing about your success.

Please write to me or email me. Nothing brightens my day more than hearing: "I did it, I lost the weight!"

I love that more than you can imagine. What we have done is planted some pretty powerful seeds in your mind.

It is interesting that when you buy a packet of seeds, the picture on the outside never looks like the seeds inside. But you have faith, so you plant the seeds in healthy soil. You position them so that they can bask in the sun and absorb the rich sunlight. Then you water them and tend to them daily. You surround this special area with a small fence to protect it from harm. And you pull the nasty weeds that spout out of nowhere. Days – weeks may go by where you think, "This isn't working." But you continue to protect, water, weed, and feed your seeds. Then one morning you look out and there is a sprout, you get excited, then another day passes, then another, until one day there is a blossom. Then it happens, the flowers spring up and you actually see the beautiful image just like the one on the packet! You are so excited. They are even more beautiful than the picture on the package. And you are!

Please take the time to revisit this information and apply it to your life consistently. You deserve to reap the benefits of this program, to experience a healthy and fulfilling life. You will be happy you chose to make yourself a priority. Life will improve in so many wonderful ways. My prayer for you is that you reconnect with your inner beauty and allow yourself to experience a peaceful, rich, and healthy life.

With love,

Your faithful virtual weight loss coach,

Rosa

Rosa Smith-Montanaro

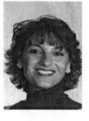

Rosa is a professional Weight Loss Coach and creator of MindOverPlatter.com, a virtual weight loss coaching community. She was named 2004 Best of the Web: eBusiness Executive of the Year.

Rosa is certified as a Success Coach and Herbal Specialist. She is certified at the master level in clinical Hypnosis, Neuro Linguistics Programming, Humanistic Neuro Linguistics Psychology, Thought Field Therapy, Time Based Techniques and Time Line Therapy TM.

Mind Over Platter® provides corporate wellness / weight management coaching and consulting to organizations and schools locally and nationally.

The focus of Rosa's work is in educating people about the power of the mind and how thoughts as well as beliefs shape reality. Rosa has developed a state of the art website MindOverPlatter.com. This is the only website of its kind. It features Rosa's entire coaching program, hypnosis sessions, seminars and materials online. She is the creator of the concept of virtual weight loss coaching combining the best of the best.

Rosa is a well–known motivational speaker. She is passionate about educating her audiences with humor, inspiration and enthusiasm.

Rosa resides in Rochester, New York with her husband and three children. She has published a variety of self-hypnosis and educational materials.

For information about ordering products or scheduling Rosa as a speaker contact: Rosa@MindOverPlatter.com or 585.227.1814

Weight Loss Coaching / Hypnosis: www.MindOverPlatter.com

References & Recommended Reading:

Unlimited Power by Tony Robbins

The Anti-Aging Zone by Barry Sears

It's Not What You're Eating, It's What's Eating You by Janet Greeson

Hypnosis for Change by Josie Hadley and Carol Staudacher

Protein Power by Michael and Mary Dan Eades

40-30-30 Fat Burning Nutrition by Joyce and Gene Daoust

Body for Life by Bill Phillips

The Carbohydrate Addict's Diet by Richard and Rachael Heller

Body Change by Montel Williams and Wini Linguvic

The Low-Carb Anti-Aging Diet by John Morgenthaler and Mia Simms

Mind Power by John Kehoe

Think Yourself Thin by Debbie Johnson

The Body Knows Diet by Caroline Sutherland

Age-Defying Diet Revolution by Dr. Atkins

The Schwarzbein Principle by Diana Schwarbein and Nancy Deville

The Seven Secrets to Slim People by Vikki Hansen and Shawn Goodman

Why Do I Eat When I'm Not Hungry? by Dr. Roger Callahan

Intuitive Eating by Evelyn Tribole and Elyse Resch

Taming the Diet Dragon by Dr. Constance C. Kirk

The Ten Habits of Naturally Slim People by Jill H. Podjasek

Diets Don't Work by Dr. Bob Schwartz.

The Metabolic Plan by Stephen Cherniske

Take Time for Your Life by Cheryl Richardson

The Power of Intention by Dr. Wayne W. Dyer

As a Man Thinketh by James Allen

The Spontaneous Fulfillment of Desire by Deepak Chopra

Your Heart's Desire by Sonia Choquette

Think and Grow Rich by Napoleon Hill

You Can Heal Your Life by Louise L. Hay

The Untold Truth Series by Wasatch Research Institute

Rosa as Your Virtual Weight Loss Coach:

Have Rosa as your personal Virtual Weight Loss Coach. www.MindOverPlatter.com is a weight loss community online that offers everything that Rosa does with her clients personally such as:

A Comprehensive Assessment that Instantly Calculates:

➢ Your Metabolism Rate

➢ Body Fat Percentage

➢ Body Mass Index

➢ How much protein, fat and carbs you need to lose weight

An Automated Food Journal

➢ Instantly calculates your calories, protein, carbs and fat

➢ Graph displaying protein, carbs and fat ratios

Daily Personally Written emails from Rosa:

➢ "Thinking Thin Thoughts" daily messages from Rosa

➢ Teleseminars / Podcasts led by Rosa

eBooks:

➢ The 21 Day-Diet™

➢ Taming the Cookie Monster Within

➢ Mind Over Platter's Weight Loss Coaching Manual

➢ Mind Over Platter's Food Journal

Digitally Recorded Seminars:

➢ The Mind Over Platter Seminar

➢ Overview of Hypnosis

➢ Tutorials of How to use MindOverPlatter.com

Digitally Recorded Hypnosis Sessions Online:

➢ Imagine Yourself Thin

➢ Imagine Yourself Enjoying Exercise

➢ Hypnotic Visualizations

Use this coupon to receive:

$22.00 off Membership to www.MindOverPlatter.com Virtual Weight Loss Coaching Program

Free Upgrade to Lifetime Status

To redeem go to: www.MindOverPlatterBook.com

Or www.MindOverPlatter.com under "What's New"